OFFICE OF POPULATION CENSUSES

COMMUNICABLE DISEASE SURVEILL

OF THE PUBLIC HEALTH LABORATO

C000077107

Series MB2 no. 17

Communicable disease statistics

statistical tables, 1990

London: HMSO

© *Crown copyright 1992*
First published 1992

ISBN 0 11 691445 9

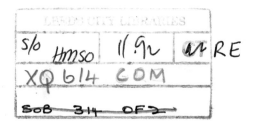

Standing order service

Placing a standing order with HMSO BOOKS enables a customer to receive future editions of this title automatically as published.

This saves the time, trouble and expense of placing individual orders and avoids the problem of knowing when to do so.

For details please write to HMSO BOOKS (PC 13A/1), Publications Centre, PO Box 276, London SW8 5DT quoting reference 02 02 043.

The standing order service also enables customers to receive automatically as published all material of their choice which additionally saves extensive catalogue research. The scope and selectivity of the service has been extended by new techniques, and there are more than 3,500 classifications to choose from. A special leaflet describing the service in detail may be obtained on request.

Contents

Introduction

Communicable disease statistics 1990 deals with statistics relating to England and Wales. Comparable statistics for earlier years and separate statistics for Scotland and Northern Ireland are published as follows:

for England and Wales for 1979 onwards in *Communicable disease statistics*, for the years 1974 to 1978 in *Statistics of infectious diseases* and for previous years in the *Registrar General's Statistical Review of England and Wales, Part I*, **Tables 28** and **34**, and **Appendices C1-C4**, **H1** and **H2**;

for Scotland - in *Scottish Health Statistics*;

for Northern Ireland - in the *Annual Report of the Registrar General for Northern Ireland*.

A summary of notifications of infectious disease for the United Kingdom and constituent countries appears in the *Annual Abstract of Statistics* issued by the Central Statistical Office.

Notification of infectious disease

Cases of infectious disease are notified by the doctor in attendance to the Proper Officer for each local government district under the Public Health Acts and Infectious Disease Regulations.

The following diseases are notifiable throughout England and Wales and reported to the Office of Population Censuses and Surveys (OPCS).

Anthrax	Malaria
Cholera	Measles
Diphtheria	Meningitis
Dysentery	Meningococcal septicaemia (without meningitis)
Acute encephalitis	
infective	Mumps
post-infectious	Ophthalmia neonatorum
Food poisoning	Paratyphoid fever
Leptospirosis	Plague

Acute poliomyelitis	Tuberculosis (all forms)
paralytic	
non-paralytic	Typhoid fever
Rabies	Typhus fever
Relapsing fever	Viral haemorrhagic fever
Rubella	
Scarlet fever	Viral hepatitis
Smallpox	Whooping cough
Tetanus	Yellow fever

The Public Health (Infectious Diseases) Regulations 1988 (Statutory Instrument: 1988 No. 1546) came into force on 1 October 1988. Under these regulations mumps and rubella became notifiable in England and Wales for the first time. 'Meningitis' replaced the term 'acute meningitis' and in addition meningococcal septicaemia (without meningitis) was added to the list of diseases to be notified. 'Infective jaundice' has been replaced by 'Viral hepatitis' and the general term 'Viral haemorrhagic fever' now includes Lassa fever and Marburg disease.

Leprosy is also notifiable and reported to the Chief Medical Officer at the Department of Health.

Prior to 1982 the Proper Officers submitted a weekly statistical return to OPCS, giving counts of the notifications that had been received during the week. This was followed at quarterly intervals by a statistical return giving extra details of the sex and age-group of the cases and incorporating any corrections to the original weekly figures.

From the beginning of 1982 a new reporting system has operated, whereby the Proper Officers continue to send in a weekly statistical summary and now also provide information about individual notifications. For example, exact age is now available rather than age-group and extra detail is provided for meningitis, tuberculosis and food poisoning. Computerisation of the individual records provides greater flexibility in analysis and enables an up-to-date count to be made at any time during the year. This system retains the provision for quarterly corrections and hence the data should be comparable with those for earlier years. Although individual records are now collected centrally, neither names nor addresses are included in the details submitted by Proper Officers. A copy of the instructions and forms used in this notification system is shown in the Appendix.

The weekly summaries of notifications are issued in the *OPCS Monitor*, Weekly Return (WR series) and are also shown, with the corrected notifications, in **Table 2** of this volume. The quarterly corrected figures are issued in the *OPCS Monitor*, Infectious diseases (MB2 series). These quarterly figures (relating to 13-week periods) form the basis of all the notification tabulations in this volume (except **Tables 2** and **13-18**), though the published quarterly figures do not always add to the published annual figures as the latter take account of late corrections. The annual figures relate to a 52-week (53 weeks in 1980 and 1986) period and not a calendar year.

Changes introduced in recent years

Tuberculosis (Tables 1a, 2-5, 8 and 10)
Tuberculosis figures for 1982 onwards may not be strictly comparable with those for earlier years because the system has been designed to enable notifications associated with chemoprophylaxis to be excluded. In the past this could only be done when chemoprophylaxis was identified on the abstract.

From 1983 onwards the specificity codes have been changed to enable pulmonary TB to be separated from other TB. Categories may not be strictly comparable with previous years but the effect is minimal.

Tables 1a and **2-5** were amended in 1982 to incorporate some of the extra data obtained through the new system of reporting notifications.

Table 1a now includes the causal organism, where known, for viral hepatitis, and whether the infection was presumed contracted abroad or in Great Britain.

Table 2 now includes original and corrected weekly notifications on one table.

Table 3 now includes rates for persons in addition to those for males and females.

Tables 3 and **4**. Figures are shown for measles by month of age up to one year and by single year of age for 1-9 years and for whooping cough by single year of age up to 9 years.

Table 5 no longer contains acute encephalitis or ophthalmia neonatorum. The data for these can be found on **Table 3** in the quarterly infectious diseases Monitors.

Tables 9 and **10**. The notification ratio, now called 'Notifications per 100 deaths' was transferred from **Table 9** to **Table 10** in 1982. It can no longer be calculated for RHAs as a comparable denominator is not available.

Base population

The population estimates used to calculate rates shown in this volume are the mid-year estimates for local government and health authority areas of England and Wales. The estimated population of an area includes all those usually resident there, whatever their nationality. Members of HM and non-UK armed forces stationed in England and Wales are included but those stationed outside are not. Students are taken to be resident at their term-time address. The estimates are updated annually by allowing for births, deaths and migration for each area. The estimates in this volume are based on the 1981 Census of Population and relate to areas with boundaries as they were defined on 1 April 1985.

Causes of death

The classification used in **Tables 1b, 6, 7** and **12** is the Ninth Revision of the *International Classification of Diseases, Injuries and Causes of Death* (ICD), which came into force in 1979.

From 1986, the number of deaths by cause excludes those at ages under 28 days. This is because a neonatal death certificate was introduced on 1 January 1986, from which it is not possible to assign an underlying cause of death. This may affect figures from 1986 in **Tables 1b, 6, 7, 11** and **12**.

Data supplied by the Communicable Disease Surveillance Centre (CDSC) of the Public Health Laboratory Service

The figures in **Tables 13** to **17** are supplied by the CDSC and are counts of laboratory identifications not necessarily associated with illness (except **Table 17**). The figures include some identifications from Northern Ireland, Eire, the Channel Islands (CI) and the Isle of Man (IOM). In **Tables 14** and **15** the number of identifications from this group is shown.

Data supplied by the Royal College of General Practitioners

The figures in **Table 18** are supplied by the Birmingham Research Unit of the Royal College of General Practitioners, and are derived from returns submitted by 60 general practices with a total population at risk of approximately 404,000. Rates are calculated by dividing the total number of newly diagnosed episodes over 13-week and 52-week periods by the average population at risk during the relevant period.

Definitions

Standard regions
The constitution of the standard regions of England and Wales in terms of counties (as constituted on 1 April 1974) is as follows:

North
Cleveland
Cumbria
Durham
Northumberland
Tyne and Wear

**Yorkshire and
  Humberside**
Humberside
North Yorkshire
South Yorkshire
West Yorkshire

East Midlands
Derbyshire
Leicestershire
Lincolnshire
Northamptonshire
Nottinghamshire

East Anglia
Cambridgeshire
Norfolk
Suffolk

South East
Bedfordshire
Berkshire
Buckinghamshire
East Sussex
Essex
Greater London
Hampshire
Hertfordshire
Isle of Wight
Kent
Oxfordshire

South East -
  continued
Surrey
West Sussex

South West
Avon
Cornwall (and Isles of
  Scilly)
Devon
Dorset
Gloucestershire
Somerset
Wiltshire

West Midlands
Hereford and
  Worcester
Shropshire
Staffordshire
Warwickshire
West Midlands

North West
Cheshire
Greater Manchester
Lancashire
Merseyside

Wales
Clwyd
Dyfed
Gwent
Gwynedd
Mid Glamorgan
Powys
South Glamorgan
West Glamorgan

Yorkshire -
  continued
Harrogate
Bradford
Airedale
Calderdale
Huddersfield
Dewsbury
Leeds Western
Leeds Eastern
Wakefield
Pontefract

Trent
North Derbyshire
Southern Derbyshire
Leicestershire
North Lincolnshire
South Lincolnshire
Bassetlaw
Central
  Nottinghamshire
Nottingham
Barnsley
Doncaster
Rotherham
Sheffield

East Anglian
Cambridge
Peterborough
West Suffolk
East Suffolk
Norwich
Great Yarmouth and
  Waveney
West Norfolk and
  Wisbech
Huntingdon

North West Thames
North Bedfordshire
South Bedfordshire
North Hertfordshire
East Hertfordshire
North West
  Hertfordshire
South West
  Hertfordshire
Barnet
Harrow
Hillingdon
Hounslow and
  Spelthorne
Ealing
Parkside
Riverside

North East Thames
Basildon and
  Thurrock
Mid Essex
North East Essex
West Essex
Southend
Barking, Havering
  and Brentwood
Hampstead
Bloomsbury
Islington
City and Hackney
Newham
Tower Hamlets
Enfield
Haringey
Redbridge
Waltham Forest

South East Thames
Brighton
Eastbourne
Hastings
South East Kent
Canterbury and
  Thanet
Dartford and
  Gravesham
Maidstone
Medway
Tunbridge Wells
Bexley
Greenwich
Bromley
West Lambeth
Camberwell
Lewisham and
  North Southwark

South West Thames
North West Surrey
West Surrey and
  North East
  Hampshire
South West Surrey
Mid Surrey
East Surrey
Chichester
Mid Downs
Worthing
Croydon
Kingston and Esher
Richmond, Twickenham
  and Roehampton
Wandsworth
Merton and Sutton

Regional health authorities

The constitution of the regional health authorities of
England and Wales in terms of district health authorities is
as follows:

Northern
Hartlepool
North Tees
South Tees
East Cumbria
South Cumbria
West Cumbria
Darlington
Durham
North West Durham
South West Durham
Northumberland
Gateshead
Newcastle

Northern -
  continued
North Tyneside
South Tyneside
Sunderland

Yorkshire
Hull
East Yorkshire
Grimsby
Scunthorpe
Northallerton
York
Scarborough

Wessex
East Dorset
West Dorset
Portsmouth and South
 East Hampshire
Southampton and
 South West
 Hampshire
Winchester
Basingstoke and
 North Hampshire
Salisbury
Swindon
Bath
Isle of Wight

Oxford
East Berkshire
West Berkshire
Aylesbury Vale
Wycombe
Milton Keynes
Kettering
Northampton
Oxfordshire

South Western
Bristol and Weston
Frenchay
Southmead
Cornwall and
 Isles of Scilly
Exeter
North Devon
Plymouth
Torbay
Cheltenham and
 District
Gloucester
Somerset

West Midlands
Bromsgrove and
 Redditch
Herefordshire
Kidderminster and
 District
Worcester and
 District
Shropshire
Mid Staffordshire
North Staffordshire
South East
 Staffordshire
Rugby
North Warwickshire
South Warwickshire
Central Birmingham
East Birmingham
North Birmingham

West Midlands -
 continued
South Birmingham
West Birmingham
Coventry
Dudley
Sandwell
Solihull
Walsall
Wolverhampton

Mersey
Chester
Crewe
Halton
Macclesfield
Warrington
Liverpool
St Helens and
 Knowsley
Southport and Formby
South Sefton
Wirral

North Western
Lancaster
Blackpool, Wyre and
 Fylde
Preston
Blackburn, Hyndburn
 and Ribble Valley
Burnley, Pendle and
 Rossendale
West Lancashire
Chorley and South
 Ribble
Bolton
Bury
North Manchester
Central Manchester
South Manchester
Oldham
Rochdale
Salford
Stockport
Tameside and Glossop
Trafford
Wigan

Wales
Clwyd
East Dyfed
Pembrokeshire
Gwent
Gwynedd
Mid Glamorgan
Powys
South Glamorgan
West Glamorgan

The reorganisation of health areas means that RHA boundaries for 1982 onwards do not always correspond exactly with local government areas, as did the statutorily defined boundaries of the old RHAs. Therefore the statistics for 1982 onwards are not always comparable with earlier years. The composition of the restructured RHAs in terms of old statutory RHAs and county districts was listed in *Communicable Disease Statistics 1983*, Series MB2 no.10.

Tables **4** and **5** show notifications of infectious diseases for RHAs and local government districts. The local government figures have been summed to the appropriate RHA but strict comparability is not always possible as five local government districts are split between RHAs. These districts have been allocated to RHAs as shown below:

Local government district	Split between RHAs:	Allocated to RHA:
High Peak	Trent North Western	Trent
Westminster, City of	North West Thames North East Thames	North West Thames
Hart	South West Thames Wessex	South West Thames
Wansdyke	Wessex South Western	Wessex
Mendip	South Western Wessex	South Western

Symbols and conventions used

-    nil

..   not available or not appropriate

Rates calculated from fewer than 20 deaths are distinguished by italic type as a warning to the user that their reliability as a measure may be affected by the small number of events.

Commentary

Measles

Until the introduction of the combined measles, mumps and rubella vaccine (MMR) in October 1988, the number of notifications of measles peaked in the Summers of two out of every three years. However, the trough of 1987 was followed by a single peak of 86,001 in 1988. In 1989 only 26,222 cases were notified and in 1990 this number declined to 13,302 (**Table 1a**). Newly diagnosed episodes of measles reported from general practitioners to the RCGP Research Unit in Birmingham show the same decrease in numbers (**Table 18**).

Following an increase in the number of children immunised, from 53 per cent in 1980 to nearly 90 per cent in 1990/91, the proportion of the total number of notifications which were for children aged under one year increased from less than 9 per cent between 1980 and 1988, to 16 per cent in 1989 and 22 per cent in 1990. However, the proportion aged 15-24 years also increased from between 3.1 and 3.7 per cent in 1986-1989 to 5.4 per cent in 1990. During the first half of the year, a large number of cases (341) were notified in South Tyneside (Tyne and Wear) (**Table 5**).

There was only one death for which measles was stated to be the cause in 1990, compared with 16 in 1988 and 3 in 1989 (**Table 1b**).

Mumps and rubella

Mumps and rubella became notifiable in October 1988 when the MMR vaccine became available. Reports to the RCGP Research Unit suggest that upsurges of mumps have occurred every three years in the past, the last being in 1987. However, the expected upsurge in 1990 did not take place. There were 79 per cent fewer notifications of mumps in 1990 (4,277) than in 1989 (**Table 1a**). Rates were highest among four year olds (**Table 3**).

Since 1986, the annual number of reports of rubella to the RCGP Research Unit has shown a steady decrease year after year. This is reflected in a reduction in the number of notifications of 53 per cent between 1989 and 1990, when there were 11,491 (**Table 1a**). Rates were highest among children aged under two years (**Table 3**).

Whooping cough

Since the mid-1970s the number of notifications of whooping cough has peaked every four years. However, since 1982 these peaks have diminished from 65,812 in that year, to 36,506 in 1986, and to 15,286 in 1990 (**Table 1a**). This decrease coincided with an increase of pertussis immunisa-

tion uptake from 30 per cent for children born in 1976 to 78 per cent for children having their second birthday in 1989/90. The proportion of all notifications which were for children under two years of age fell from 24 per cent in 1978 to 18 per cent in 1990 (**Table 4**).

In spite of the decrease in the number of cases notified, there were more deaths for which whooping cough (ICD 033) was stated to be the cause in 1990 (7) than in 1986, when there were 3 (**Table 1b**). All seven children were under four months of age.

Tuberculosis

While the number of notifications increased by 5 per cent between 1988 and 1989, there was a small decline of 4 per cent from 5,432 to 5,204 in 1990. Notifications of respiratory tuberculosis fell from 4,146 in 1989 to 3,942 in 1990 (**Table 1a**). While there was no great regional difference in the change between 1989 and 1990, there were small increases in East Anglia, Yorkshire and Humberside, and North West standard regions, and decreases in all other regions and in Greater London (**Table 5**). There were 390 deaths in 1990 for which tuberculosis (ICD 010-018) (excluding late effects) was stated as the cause. This was a decrease of 12 per cent compared with 1989 (**Table 1b**).

Meningococcal meningitis

The number of notifications of meningococcal meningitis increased steadily from 401 in 1984 to 1,304 in 1988. After a small decline in 1989, the number did not change appreciably between 1989 and 1990 when there were 1,138 (**Table 1a**). This was largely due to an increase in the number notified during nine of the first ten weeks of 1990 compared with 1989. During years when a large number of cases occur, the number begins to increase sharply during the last six weeks of the year to peak in early January. At the end of 1990, however, the increase was very much smaller and started later than in 1989 (**Table 2**). As in previous years, rates in 1990 were highest among children aged less than two years. There was, however, an increase in the number of notifications of meningococcal septicaemia (without meningitis) from 229 in 1989 to 277 in 1990 (**Table 1a**). These occurred in highest numbers during the first few weeks of 1990 (**Table 2**).

As in earlier years of this current upsurge, the infection was widespread, with at least one case of meningococcal meningitis or meningococcal septicaemia (without meningitis) being notified in 321 of the 403 districts in England and Wales (**Table 5**). However, more than 20 notifications were reported from five densely populated districts, Birmingham (39) and Coventry (22) in West Midlands, Liverpool (27) and Wirral (22) in Merseyside, and Manchester (22) in Greater Manchester.

There were 169 deaths for which meningococcal infection (ICD 036) was stated as the cause in 1990 (**Table 1b**). Of these, 48 (28 per cent) were to children aged between 28 days and one year. Twice as many boys in this age-group died from this infection as girls.

Neisseria meningitidis was the most common organism associated with meningitis and/or encephalitis reported by laboratories to CDSC in 1990. Of these reports, 25 per cent were from children aged less than one year (**Table 17**).

Viral hepatitis
In 1969, the first full year during which infective jaundice was notifiable, 23,580 cases were reported. This number fell to 3,216 in 1979 before increasing again to 10,605 in 1982. Over the following five years, the number again decreased to 3,379 in 1987, but in subsequent years increased again gradually to 9,005 in 1990 (**Table 1a**). In 1990, 92 per cent of cases for which the cause was stated were due to hepatitis A. The increase in 1990 compared with 1987 was entirely due to an increase in the number of cases notified as due to hepatitis A, which increased fourfold, and to a smaller extent for cases for which the cause was not known. Of cases due to hepatitis A, 95 per cent in 1990 were presumed contracted in Great Britain, representing an increase of 80 per cent compared with 1987. The number stated to have been contracted abroad increased from 200 in 1987 to 302 in 1990 (**Table 1a**). Areas reporting large numbers of notifications include Bradford, Calderdale, Leeds and Kirklees in West Yorkshire, and the adjacent areas of Hartlepool and Stockton on Tees in Cleveland, from Corby in Northamptonshire, from Shepway in Kent and from Liverpool in Merseyside (**Table 5**). Large numbers were reported from West Yorkshire in 1988 and 1989. As in 1987, highest rates in 1990 occurred among 5-14 year olds and these age-groups showed a larger increase than among other age-groups (**Table 3**).

There were 26 per cent fewer reports of hepatitis B antigen from laboratories to CDSC in 1990 (1,904) than in 1987, confirming that hepatitis B did not contribute to the upsurge in viral hepatitis occurring between 1987 and 1990 (**Table 13**).

Food poisoning
In 1990, for the first year since 1985, the number of notifications of food poisoning did not increase compared with the previous year. However, the total number of cases either notified or ascertained by other means declined by only 1 per cent to 52,145 in 1990 compared with 1989. This small decrease was almost entirely due to a fall in the number of people stated to have acquired their infection

abroad (**Table 1a**). Three districts reported over a thousand notifications, Leeds (1,590) and Bradford (1,039) in West Yorkshire and Sheffield (1,064) in South Yorkshire. Six other districts (Kirklees in West Yorkshire, Birmingham, Coventry and Dudley in West Midlands, Bolton in Greater Manchester and Cardiff in South Glamorgan) reported more than 600 cases, and a further three districts (Barnet in Greater London, Bristol in Avon and Wirral in Merseyside) reported more than 500 cases (**Table 5**). Highest rates for all cases reported were for adults aged 15-44 years (**Table 3**).

Since 1985, the total number of identifications of salmonellas reported by laboratories to CDSC has increased each year. In 1990 there were 26,203 reports compared with 12,270 in 1985. Until 1987 the serotype most frequently reported was *S.typhimurium*. However, the number of reports of *S.enteritidis* increased steadily from 1,568 in 1984 to 16,002 in 1990, and surpassed the number of reports of *S.typhimurium* in 1988 (**Table 15**). The largest number of reports of salmonellas were received from Yorkshire; 64 per cent of those were *S.enteritidis* (**Table 15**).

Dysentery
Since 1988, the number of notifications of dysentery has declined by 25 per cent from 3,692 in that year to 2,756 in 1990 (**Table 1a**). Highest numbers were reported from Leeds (288) in West Yorkshire, Cardiff (151) in South Glamorgan and Bristol (126) in Avon (**Table 5**). Notification rates were highest among one year olds (**Table 3**).

The number of identifications of shigellas reported from laboratories to CDSC also decreased, from 3,664 in 1988 to 3,405 in 1990. Of the 1990 total, 18 per cent were reported from laboratories in Yorkshire RHA (**Table 15**). Of all shigellas reported, 71 per cent were *S.sonnei*.

Typhoid and paratyphoid fevers
The total numbers of notifications of typhoid and paratyphoid fevers has varied little since 1980, with the exception of 1988 when a large number of cases of paratyphoid occurred among people who had attended a function in the West Midlands. During 1990, there was a small increase in the number of notifications of paratyphoid acquired in Great Britain (**Table 1a**). An outbreak occurred in the North of England involving 12 people, none of whom had a history of recent foreign travel. A new phage type was identified from these patients (Taunton var 2). A worker in a butcher's shop was identified as the source.

Malaria
Between 1985 and 1987, the number of notifications of malaria decreased by 29 per cent, from 1,695 to 1,202. Since 1987, however, the number has increased each year to 1,493 in 1990 (**Table 1a**). In 1990, 872 (58 per cent) of notifications were reported from the South East standard

region, 693 (46 per cent of the total) of which were from Greater London. Districts within London with the highest number were Brent (90), Hackney (41), Camden (40), Newham (38), and Westminster (38). Other districts from which a relatively large number were reported were Birmingham (48) and Bradford (45) (**Table 5**).

Table 1a   Notifications of selected infectious diseases, 1980 to 1990   **England and Wales**

Final numbers after correction (including original cases in port health authorities)

Disease	1980	1981	1982	1983	1984	1985	1986	1987	1988	1989	1990
Cholera	4	9	1	5	3	7	9	3	17	13	19
Typhoid fever	211	184	166	183	152	178	156	140	174	164	178
presumed contracted											
in Great Britain	29	18	27	16	32	20	21	20	22	15	22
abroad ⎱	182	166	126	146	104	140	120	95	117	114	123
not stated ⎰			13	21	16	18	15	25	35	35	33
Paratyphoid fever	79	70	69	78	70	75	84	63	180	88	93
presumed contracted											
abroad	65	58	53	57	54	62	65	46	52	60	64
in Great Britain ⎱	14	12	8	16	4	5	10	7	115	7	13
not stated ⎰			8	5	12	8	9	10	13	21	16
Dysentery	2,709	3,401	2,850	5,004	6,844	5,335	4,774	3,617	3,692	3,278	2,756
presumed contracted											
abroad	..	..	..	..	..	..	..	767	740	686	592
in Great Britain	..	..	..	..	..	..	..	2,165	2,254	2,011	1,489
not stated	..	..	..	..	..	..	..	685	698	581	675
Food poisoning	..	..	14,253	17,735	20,702	19,242	23,948	29,331	39,713	52,557	52,145
Formally notified	10,318	9,936	9,964	12,273	13,247	13,143	16,502	20,363	27,826	38,086	36,945
presumed contracted											
abroad	..	..	927	1,071	1,138	1,089	1,431	1,757	1,939	1,990	1,612
in Great Britain	..	..	7,487	9,209	10,303	9,909	12,347	14,295	18,689	24,896	24,353
not stated	..	..	1,550	1,993	1,806	2,145	2,724	4,311	7,198	11,200	10,980
Ascertained by other means	..	..	4,289	5,462	7,455	6,099	7,446	8,968	11,887	14,471	15,200
presumed contracted											
abroad	..	..	424	607	695	662	856	1,128	1,352	1,238	915
in Great Britain	..	..	3,149	3,842	5,532	4,335	5,023	5,761	7,789	10,613	11,031
not stated	..	..	716	1,013	1,228	1,102	1,567	2,079	2,746	2,620	3,254
Tuberculosis†	9,145	8,128	7,410 *	6,803 *	6,141 *	5,857 *	5,993 *	5,086 *	5,164 *	5,432 *	5,204 *
Respiratory	6,673	5,859	5,826	5,318	4,871	4,660	4,759	4,010	4,022	4,146	3,942
Pulmonary lesion (with or without mediastinal nodes and/or pleural effusion)	..	..	5,326	4,785	4,494	4,247	4,298	3,603	3,629	3,777	3,572
Mediastinal nodes and/or a pleural effusion without a pulmonary lesion	..	..	352	423	330	364	407	367	339	328	323
Pulmonary lesion and meningitis	..	..	..	13	4	2	11	4	12	2	6
Pulmonary lesion and other forms	..	..	..	82	37	44	36	33	34	37	40
Mediastinal nodes and meningitis	..	..	..	1	1	1	-	-	2	-	-
Mediastinal nodes and other forms	..	..	..	14	5	2	7	3	6	2	1
Meningitis with or without other forms	..	..	..	71	57	50	71	50	59	50	75
Other forms alone	..	..	1,512	1,414	1,213	1,147	1,163	1,026	1,083	1,236	1,187
Plague	-	-	-	-	-	-	-	-	-	-	-
Anthrax	-	-	1	-	2	2	1	-	2	1	2
Diphtheria	5	2	4	4	4	4	4	2	1	2	2
Whooping cough	21,131	19,395	65,812	19,340	5,517	22,046	36,506	15,203	5,117	11,646	15,286
Scarlet fever	11,118	7,148	7,601	6,539	6,327	6,438	6,888	6,439	5,949	8,295	7,187
Meningitis Ø	1,796	1,393	1,272	1,226	1,230	1,533	2,172	2,542	2,987	2,722	2,572
meningococcal	509	464	410	428	401	550	870	1,080	1,304	1,133	1,138
pneumococcal			87	74	78	82	143	136	209	174	156
influenzal (Haemophilus influenzae)			177	173	217	206	268	354	436	470	431
viral	1,287	929	321	308	244	323	450	493	490	397	353
other specified			132	106	141	186	209	234	295	270	227
unspecified			145	137	149	186	232	245	253	278	267
Meningococcal septicaemia ≠ (without meningitis)	..	..	..	..	..	..	..	..	...	229	277
Tetanus	18	15	12	6	6	12	11	9	12	16	9
Acute poliomyelitis	3	2	2	4	-	4	3	3	2	1	1
paralytic	2	2	2	4	-	3	2	3	1	1	1
non-paralytic	1	-	-	-	-	1	1	-	1	-	-
Smallpox	-	-	-	-	-	-	-	-	-	-	-

*   Excluding chemoprophylaxis.
†   See note on page vi.
Ø   Acute meningitis was redesignated meningitis on 1 October 1988.
≠   Became notifiable on 1 October 1988.

Table 1a - *continued*

Disease	1980	1981	1982	1983	1984	1985	1986	1987	1988	1989	1990
Measles	139,487	52,979	94,200	103,703	62,080	97,408	82,061	42,165	86,001	26,222	13,302
Rubella ≠	..	..	..	..	..	..	..	..	..	24,570	11,491
Yellow fever	-	-	-	-	-	-	-	-	-	-	-
Acute encephalitis	91	58	71	56	37	39	51	57	65	40	39
infective	43	30	25	31	22	24	28	29	36	28	32
post-infectious	48	28	46	25	15	15	23	28	29	12	7
Viral hepatitis Ø	5,143	9,841	10,605	6,316	5,805	4,382	3,630	3,379	5,063	7,071	9,005
hepatitis A	..	..	..	..	..	..	..	1,836	3,190	5,278	7,316
presumed contracted											
abroad	..	..	..	..	..	..	..	200	267	256	302
in Great Britain	..	..	..	..	..	..	..	1,126	1,945	3,431	5,515
not stated	..	..	..	..	..	..	..	510	978	1,591	1,499
hepatitis B	..	..	..	..	..	..	..	444	390	432	435
presumed contracted											
abroad	..	..	..	..	..	..	..	42	28	46	35
in Great Britain	..	..	..	..	..	..	..	269	231	230	239
not stated	..	..	..	..	..	..	..	133	131	156	161
hepatitis 'non A - non B'	..	..	..	..	..	..	..	249	363	256	169
presumed contracted											
abroad	..	..	..	..	..	..	..	41	34	15	4
in Great Britain	..	..	..	..	..	..	..	135	245	78	55
not stated	..	..	..	..	..	..	..	73	84	163	110
hepatitis other/not known	..	..	..	..	..	..	..	850	1,120	1,105	1,085
presumed contracted											
abroad	..	..	..	..	..	..	..	29	37	29	21
in Great Britain	..	..	..	..	..	..	..	297	442	463	369
not stated	..	..	..	..	..	..	..	524	641	613	695
Rabies	-	1	-	-	-	-	1	1	1	-	-
Mumps ≠	..	..	..	..	..	..	..	..	..	20,713	4,277
Viral haemorrhagic fever Ω	-	-	-	-	-	-	-	-	-	-	2
Typhus fever	4	5	1	6	3	2	6	8	1	7	4
Malaria	1,296	1,278	1,183	1,125	1,398	1,695	1,663	1,202	1,271	1,478	1,493
Relapsing fever	1	1	-	-	1	1	-	-	-	-	2
Ophthalmia neonatorum	278	210	201	208	247	258	298	300	374	427	440
Leptospirosis	13	23	14	23	19	31	22	25	36	32	20

≠ Became notifiable on 1 October 1988.
Ø Infective jaundice was redesignated viral hepatitis on 1 October 1988.
Ω From 1 October 1988, viral haemorrhagic fever includes Marburg disease and Lassa fever.

Table 1b   Deaths from selected infectious diseases, 1980 to 1990   **England and Wales**

ICD number	Cause of death	1980	1981	1982	1983	1984	1985	1986	1987	1988	1989	1990
001-139	**Infectious and parasitic diseases**	**2,239**	**2,102**	**2,116**	**2,043**	**2,295**	**2,381**	**2,470**	**2,375**	**2,480**	**2,543**	**2,446**
001-009	**Intestinal infectious diseases**	**186**	**194**	**206**	**177**	**193**	**177**	**176**	**162**	**164**	**185**	**187**
001	Cholera	-	-	-	1	-	1	-	-	-	-	-
002.0	Typhoid fever	1	2	3	1	-	-	-	2	1	-	2
002.1-002.9	Paratyphoid fever	-	-	-	-	-	-	-	-	-	-	-
003	Other salmonella infections	37	34	65	49	54	49	40	52	58	61	68
004	Shigellosis	4	6	2	4	2	2	3	3	2	1	-
005	Other food poisoning (bacterial)	2	1	-	-	1	-	3	3	2	2	1
006,007	Amoebiasis and other protozoal intestinal diseases	1	2	2	-	1	1	2	1	-	2	4
008	Intestinal infections due to other organisms	30	22	35	28	31	39	52	26	36	54	43
009	Ill-defined intestinal infections	111	127	99	91	104	85	76	75	65	65	69
010-018	**Tuberculosis**	**605**	**557**	**564**	**467**	**490**	**523**	**471**	**430**	**478**	**443**	**390**
011	Pulmonary tuberculosis	471	430	450	371	375	407	373	325	382	330	309
013	Tuberculosis of meninges and central nervous system	26	26	22	15	30	18	15	20	13	22	13
013.0	Tuberculous meningitis	24	23	18	15	28	17	12	20	9	19	12
010-018 Rem	Tuberculosis, other forms	108	101	92	81	85	98	83	85	83	91	68
020-027	**Zoonotic bacterial diseases**	**5**	**8**	**3**	**13**	**7**	**7**	**11**	**17**	**11**	**18**	**11**
027.0	Listeriosis	5	7	3	13	6	7	11	17	11	16	9
030-041	**Other bacterial diseases**	**473**	**550**	**597**	**516**	**593**	**700**	**822**	**881**	**909**	**984**	**952**
032	Diphtheria	-	-	1	-	-	-	-	-	-	-	-
033	Whooping cough	6	5	14	5	1	4	3	5	-	1	7
034,035	Streptococcal sore throat, scarlatina and erysipelas	5	8	5	4	5	2	3	10	5	7	1
036	Meningococcal infection	71	85	70	70	79	97	141	155	174	203	169
036.0	Meningococcal meningitis	26	28	20	20	26	36	44	37	45	53	39
036.2	Meningococcaemia	33	40	34	40	47	46	75	101	105	133	116
036.3	Waterhouse-Friderichsen syndrome, meningococcal	8	15	15	10	6	14	20	16	22	14	11
037	Tetanus	4	6	1	1	3	3	3	2	5	2	1
038	Septicaemia	359	416	472	401	470	550	613	661	669	715	711
038.0	Streptococcal septicaemia	13	28	15	20	36	28	23	31	23	28	31
038.1	Staphylococcal septicaemia	35	39	55	37	55	69	74	64	73	53	71
038.2	Pneumococcal septicaemia	10	15	12	11	11	15	15	10	18	17	22
038.3-038.9	Other and unspecified septicaemias	301	334	390	333	368	438	501	556	555	617	587
039	Actinomycotic infections	4	4	2	4	6	7	1	1	5	4	1
040.0	Gas gangrene	6	11	10	8	6	6	9	8	6	3	4
045-049	**Poliomyelitis and other non-arthropod-borne viral diseases of central nervous system**	**102**	**101**	**71**	**80**	**97**	**96**	**95**	**95**	**90**	**95**	**99**
046	Slow virus infection of central nervous system	34	40	31	27	54	46	40	46	40	43	45
046.1	Jakob-Creutzfeldt disease	25	31	23	23	42	35	29	30	34	30	38
046.2	Subacute sclerosing panencephalitis	7	9	8	3	10	8	7	10	5	7	2
047,048	Meningitis due to enterovirus and other enterovirus diseases of central nervous system	16	14	5	17	11	4	4	6	9	17	15
050-057	**Viral diseases accompanied by exanthem**	**178**	**109**	**117**	**128**	**188**	**191**	**184**	**161**	**164**	**165**	**137**
052	Chickenpox	31	16	23	23	26	25	25	24	30	19	24
053	Herpes zoster	78	45	57	64	121	116	111	103	98	110	88
054	Herpes simplex	42	33	23	24	31	39	37	27	20	33	24
055	Measles	26	15	13	16	10	11	10	6	16	3	1
056	Rubella	-	-	1	1	-	-	1	1	-	-	-
060-066	**Arthropod-borne viral diseases**	**-**	**-**	**1**	**-**	**-**	**-**	**-**	**-**	**-**	**-**	**-**
070-079	**Other diseases due to viruses and chlamydiae**	**164**	**154**	**139**	**185**	**182**	**139**	**164**	**166**	**181**	**180**	**197**

Note: Annual figures should be compared with caution because: i. The Ninth Revision of the ICD was introduced on 1 January 1979 (see MB2 no.12, page 2). ii. A change in the coding instructions (WHO Rule 3) was introduced on 1 January 1984 (see MB2 no.11, page 2). iii. From 1986 neonatal deaths by cause are excluded (see note on page vi).

Table 1b - *continued*

ICD number	Cause of death	1980	1981	1982	1983	1984	1985	1986	1987	1988	1989	1990
070	Viral hepatitis	97	99	85	114	107	72	91	109	106	102	112
070.0-070.1	Viral hepatitis A	21	27	22	18	11	12	10	10	12	6	14
070.2-070.3	Viral hepatitis B	35	35	32	56	69	44	57	69	59	58	53
072	Mumps	2	4	2	4	3	2	4	3	2	1	-
075	Infectious mononucleosis	4	2	2	5	11	2	2	4	6	3	2
078.5	Cytomegalic inclusion disease	2	4	5	7	7	11	10	8	10	13	26
080-088	**Rickettsioses and other arthropod-borne diseases**	**8**	**3**	**10**	**8**	**6**	**7**	**4**	**11**	**7**	**5**	**5**
084	Malaria	8	2	10	7	4	5	3	7	6	4	3
090-099	**Syphilis and other venereal diseases**	**60**	**55**	**46**	**49**	**68**	**40**	**42**	**35**	**30**	**19**	**18**
100-104	**Other spirochaetal diseases**	**5**	**3**	**2**	**2**	**-**	**4**	**1**	**1**	**5**	**3**	**3**
100	Leptospirosis	4	1	2	2	-	3	1	1	5	2	3
110-118	**Mycoses**	**26**	**44**	**34**	**35**	**32**	**57**	**47**	**42**	**45**	**41**	**48**
112	Candidiases	8	9	6	10	11	13	11	13	10	9	15
117.3	Aspergillosis	17	30	23	21	15	38	26	27	29	26	28
120-129	**Helminthiases**	**5**	**4**	**8**	**4**	**4**	**7**	**2**	**6**	**5**	**8**	**9**
130-136	**Other infectious and parasitic diseases**	**91**	**80**	**98**	**110**	**122**	**137**	**137**	**141**	**120**	**149**	**161**
130	Toxoplasmosis	-	2	-	4	2	1	2	-	6	10	7
135	Sarcoidosis	62	64	75	80	84	98	89	90	86	89	88
137-139	**Late effects of infectious and parasitic diseases**	**331**	**240**	**220**	**269**	**313**	**296**	**314**	**227**	**271**	**248**	**229**
137	Late effects of tuberculosis	298	207	186	232	263	251	262	195	240	206	187
138	Late effects of acute poliomyelitis	21	24	19	21	38	29	33	21	24	29	35
320-326	**Inflammatory diseases of central nervous system (excluding those infections included in ICD 001-139)**	**399**	**400**	**403**	**380**	**366**	**426**	**381**	**359**	**321**	**344**	**298**
320-322	Meningitis	277	266	286	281	246	306	271	260	230	246	203
320	Bacterial meningitis	198	176	184	206	178	229	181	196	165	185	147
320.0	Haemophilus meningitis	20	14	30	24	23	31	24	23	20	23	26
320.1	Pneumococcal meningitis	72	66	72	78	65	88	75	70	79	82	60
320.2	Streptococcal meningitis	19	16	19	19	23	27	15	20	5	12	7
320.3	Staphylococcal meningitis	3	3	6	7	5	6	5	5	5	4	5
460-466	**Acute respiratory infections (except pneumonia and influenza)**	**1,105**	**1,024**	**1,085**	**959**	**854**	**975**	**934**	**732**	**786**	**800**	**673**
466	Acute bronchitis and bronchiolitis	983	912	981	872	786	901	840	641	697	697	599
480-486	**Pneumonia**	**53,704**	**54,057**	**56,529**	**55,513**	**24,687**	**27,931**	**27,624**	**24,603**	**26,424**	**28,777**	**26,817**
480	Viral pneumonia	342	309	373	326	249	278	272	137	169	184	171
481	Pneumococcal pneumonia	2,428	2,312	2,518	2,376	2,415	2,516	2,256	2,011	2,213	2,391	2,185
482	Other bacterial pneumonia	109	104	139	133	150	161	141	110	137	134	134
487	**Influenza**	**514**	**626**	**716**	**796**	**346**	**662**	**587**	**190**	**285**	**2,114**	**791**
487.0	Influenza with pneumonia	390	465	497	577	248	477	410	116	182	1,472	571
771	**Infections specific to the perinatal period**	**96**	**85**	**81**	**84**	**103**	**93**	**3**	**6**	**10**	**6**	**10**
771.0	Congenital rubella	-	1	-	4	5	-	-	2	-	3	1
771.1	Congenital cytomegalovirus infection	4	3	2	2	4	10	1	2	5	3	3
771.2	Other congenital infections	6	3	10	8	3	7	1	2	4	-	3

Note: Annual figures should be compared with caution because: i. The Ninth Revision of the ICD was introduced on 1 January 1979 (see MB2 no.12, page 2). ii. A change in the coding instructions (WHO Rule 3) was introduced on 1 January 1984 (see MB2 no.11, page 2). iii. From 1986 neonatal deaths by cause are excluded (see note on page vi).

Table 2 Series MB2 no 17

Table 2 Weekly notifications of selected infectious diseases and deaths from selected causes, 1990
a original
b corrected

England and Wales

Week ended		Notifications (including port health authorities)													
		Typhoid fever		Paratyphoid fever		Dysentery (amoebic and bacillary)		Food poisoning formally notified		Food poisoning ascertained by other means		All tuberculosis*†		Whooping cough	
		a	b	a	b	a	b	a	b	a	b	a	b	a	b
January	5	4	4	1	-	40	35	376	360	139	128	90	90	269	269
	12	2	2	2	2	46	46	451	426	169	149	97	95	276	276
	19	1	1	-	-	55	55	467	455	228	217	111	109	273	273
	26	3	3	1	1	51	50	422	409	265	249	98	97	345	345
February	2	3	3	1	1	60	58	473	455	178	167	101	101	304	303
	9	3	3	2	2	49	48	472	459	244	169	103	103	374	373
	16	2	2	2	1	52	48	505	496	182	162	131	130	395	394
	23	3	3	3	3	41	40	492	476	213	191	104	104	322	322
March	2	5	5	-	-	36	36	477	457	242	225	93	91	260	260
	9	2	1	1	1	51	49	527	507	213	197	105	103	286	285
	16	2	2	4	4	43	45	536	500	235	219	115	112	321	324
	23	3	3	2	2	45	41	466	449	221	204	101	100	297	297
	30	3	2	4	4	44	44	469	445	219	193	87	84	332	332
April	6	3	3	1	1	31	25	506	488	177	160	119	119	311	309
	13	1	1	2	2	32	32	383	376	170	155	92	90	225	223
	20	1	1	4	4	27	25	436	430	141	132	93	91	260	259
	27	3	3	2	2	42	42	555	520	213	197	121	119	315	314
May	4	5	5	-	-	55	53	529	505	221	205	129	127	274	274
	11	1	1	3	2	46	45	533	511	217	200	93	92	277	277
	18	3	3	-	-	65	57	770	750	331	302	125	121	356	355
	25	3	3	1	1	60	58	1,032	989	310	285	120	119	375	375
June	1	4	5	-	-	51	51	760	731	276	258	62	59	277	277
	8	3	3	-	-	56	56	1,061	1,033	389	357	86	86	330	330
	15	2	2	3	3	54	53	962	936	348	323	115	116	338	338
	22	9	9	3	3	45	45	856	835	359	341	109	105	361	358
	29	5	4	2	2	50	49	969	939	366	345	117	115	354	353
July	6	1	1	2	2	33	33	849	837	385	366	118	118	313	311
	13	3	3	2	2	47	45	819	808	434	404	120	115	381	380
	20	1	1	4	4	36	36	897	883	330	319	107	107	322	322
	27	7	7	2	2	60	58	1,165	1,162	377	352	119	117	284	283
August	3	2	2	1	1	49	48	970	959	436	407	128	128	277	277
	10	5	4	-	-	43	42	986	981	503	469	117	115	306	306
	17	8	8	-	-	62	64	1,209	1,207	506	470	120	114	381	378
	24	3	3	2	2	59	59	1,087	1,094	512	456	111	110	411	410
	31	5	6	-	-	69	69	851	850	413	386	59	60	338	337
September	7	9	9	1	1	80	77	1,272	1,228	618	584	100	98	453	452
	14	3	3	2	2	78	78	1,187	1,177	567	523	74	72	451	424
	21	7	6	3	3	77	82	1,123	1,108	491	463	101	99	378	378
	28	9	9	3	3	80	77	1,039	1,023	522	496	111	109	357	357
October	5	10	10	4	3	65	65	874	869	554	495	102	102	272	271
	12	5	5	3	3	68	67	847	829	373	353	114	115	194	194
	19	6	6	4	4	65	64	849	829	308	288	79	79	202	200
	26	3	3	2	2	78	76	760	751	366	349	98	96	150	149
November	2	1	1	1	1	55	55	820	797	378	362	105	104	189	188
	9	2	2	2	2	56	51	784	763	351	322	96	92	200	198
	16	1	1	2	2	39	37	773	731	350	330	95	96	211	208
	23	2	2	2	2	67	66	750	733	296	279	90	89	241	241
	30	2	2	3	3	63	62	689	634	302	271	91	90	255	255
December	7	3	3	-	-	78	77	520	500	219	203	79	76	203	203
	14	3	2	2	3	83	83	515	498	214	201	105	103	203	203
	21	1	1	2	2	76	75	498	484	234	229	84	75	174	174
	28	1	1	3	3	24	24	279	273	99	93	47	47	93	92
Total (52 Weeks)		**182**	**178**	**96**	**93**	**2,817**	**2,756**	**37,897**	**36,945**	**16,404**	**15,200**	**5,287**	**5,204**	**15,346**	**15,286**

*See note on page vi.
†Excluding chemoprophylaxis.

Notifications												Week ended	
Scarlet fever		Meningitis (all)		Meningitis (meningococcal)		Meningococcal septicaemia (without meningitis)		Measles		Rubella			
a	b	a	b	a	b	a	b	a	b	a	b		
155	155	100	100	63	63	9	9	204	204	174	174	5	January
125	125	114	113	69	68	17	17	215	215	144	144	12	
160	160	73	73	48	48	10	10	203	203	183	183	19	
156	156	63	64	37	37	14	12	260	260	204	204	26	
200	200	69	69	40	40	13	13	233	233	222	222	2	February
198	198	71	71	35	35	11	11	290	290	281	281	9	
216	216	69	68	39	39	3	3	318	318	258	258	16	
225	225	55	55	35	35	7	7	358	358	329	329	23	
199	199	54	54	29	29	6	6	344	344	256	256	2	March
184	183	59	59	28	28	7	7	377	377	337	337	9	
262	261	51	50	26	26	6	6	341	341	346	346	16	
279	279	59	58	22	22	7	7	325	325	363	363	23	
260	252	38	38	13	13	6	6	367	367	380	380	30	
251	251	69	69	41	41	6	6	357	357	414	414	6	April
178	178	44	44	22	22	5	5	251	251	291	291	13	
205	205	53	53	26	26	2	2	323	332	300	300	20	
192	193	43	42	22	20	13	13	372	372	333	333	27	
175	175	48	48	22	22	9	8	320	320	326	326	4	May
150	150	33	32	17	16	5	4	297	297	277	277	11	
145	144	65	65	30	31	8	7	296	296	342	342	18	
184	184	44	44	20	20	4	4	367	367	311	311	25	
122	122	36	36	17	17	8	8	221	221	234	234	1	June
108	108	52	52	25	25	6	6	292	292	222	222	8	
122	122	42	39	21	19	2	2	315	315	276	276	15	
126	125	40	40	12	12	3	3	272	272	252	252	22	
145	145	36	36	19	19	7	7	304	304	278	278	29	
192	192	39	39	13	13	8	8	314	314	331	331	6	July
128	128	49	49	13	14	3	2	286	286	286	286	13	
127	127	35	35	13	13	3	3	264	264	275	275	20	
104	104	40	40	8	8	5	5	267	267	242	242	27	
82	82	45	43	11	11	4	3	225	225	161	161	3	August
68	68	57	57	15	15	2	2	257	257	160	160	10	
46	46	44	44	11	11	4	4	234	234	157	157	17	
52	52	28	27	11	11	2	2	186	186	131	131	24	
46	46	39	39	11	10	3	3	168	168	88	88	31	
60	58	34	34	15	15	4	4	187	187	170	170	7	September
61	61	32	32	9	9	3	3	172	172	118	118	14	
58	58	26	26	9	9	2	2	169	169	132	132	21	
72	72	38	38	12	12	2	2	192	192	152	152	28	
72	72	48	47	15	14	6	6	184	184	135	135	5	October
106	106	47	46	14	14	5	5	210	210	142	142	12	
111	111	48	48	16	16	4	4	261	261	181	181	19	
93	93	35	35	10	10	4	4	203	203	133	133	26	
83	83	48	48	11	11	4	4	198	198	150	150	2	November
105	105	57	56	21	21	-	-	203	203	144	144	9	
121	122	57	57	22	22	2	2	208	208	130	130	16	
144	144	38	38	14	14	3	3	224	224	162	162	23	
109	109	38	38	17	17	1	1	188	188	153	153	30	
125	125	48	48	15	15	3	3	207	207	144	144	7	December
118	117	42	42	12	12	5	5	176	176	102	102	14	
133	133	52	52	23	22	2	2	206	206	116	116	21	
62	62	44	42	28	26	5	6	91	91	63	63	28	
7,200	7,187	2,588	2,572	1,147	1,138	283	277	13,302	13,302	11,491	11,491		Total (52 Weeks)

Table 2 Series MB2 no. 17

Table 2 - *continued*

Week ended		Notifications						Deaths≠		
		Viral hepatitis		Mumps		Malaria		Bronchitis** (acute and chronic) (ICD 466,490, 491)	Influenza and influenzal pneumonia (ICD 487)	Pneumonia†† (ICD 480-486)
		a	b	a	b	a	b			
January	5	114	114	118	118	9	9	302	357	1,486
	12	186	186	106	106	22	22	242	155	1,094
	19	145	142	90	90	29	28	177	81	824
	26	160	159	98	98	26	26	181	43	681
February	2	150	150	105	105	40	40	155	26	660
	9	178	177	119	119	24	24	151	12	638
	16	183	183	126	126	22	22	138	8	589
	23	150	148	92	92	26	26	157	2	580
March	2	139	138	112	112	15	15	94	5	521
	9	145	145	106	106	14	14	124	1	504
	16	156	157	103	103	18	18	126	-	504
	23	182	181	142	142	16	16	105	-	481
	30	179	174	106	106	18	18	114	2	455
April	6	168	163	105	105	39	35	109	2	480
	13	132	132	83	83	20	20	88	-	401
	20	129	128	86	86	9	9	128	-	517
	27	193	187	93	93	34	34	138	1	531
May	4	160	158	105	105	41	41	103	2	511
	11	158	154	65	65	12	12	92	1	435
	18	182	172	98	98	24	24	85	-	406
	25	161	160	108	108	36	36	101	-	377
June	1	151	149	71	71	13	13	85	-	410
	8	149	149	92	92	40	40	87	2	436
	15	163	161	102	102	40	40	98	-	407
	22	171	166	90	90	33	33	99	-	419
	29	154	152	94	94	50	49	90	1	422
July	6	142	142	101	101	29	29	66	2	380
	13	179	179	91	91	26	26	71	1	394
	20	168	165	88	88	42	41	84	1	428
	27	167	167	90	90	47	47	87	2	408
August	3	165	165	67	67	41	40	63	2	387
	10	154	154	59	59	50	50	72	1	430
	17	150	148	77	77	32	32	73	1	346
	24	129	129	59	59	40	40	76	1	336
	31	117	117	44	44	54	53	54	-	361
September	7	145	140	53	53	52	52	67	-	318
	14	188	186	60	60	32	32	55	-	313
	21	209	209	50	50	49	49	60	-	310
	28	209	208	61	61	34	34	83	2	346
October	5	172	172	47	47	37	37	81	-	395
	12	236	235	66	66	35	35	82	1	390
	19	242	242	71	71	30	30	79	2	419
	26	243	243	71	71	31	30	65	3	428
November	2	227	227	58	58	27	27	89	2	486
	9	234	234	66	66	26	26	81	2	425
	16	246	244	69	69	19	19	107	2	433
	23	235	229	78	78	21	21	87	3	424
	30	210	209	59	59	29	29	104	6	485
December	7	262	262	52	52	22	22	103	4	495
	14	235	234	58	58	14	14	119	11	552
	21	178	179	50	50	11	11	134	7	754
	28	102	101	17	17	3	3	119	9	695
Total (52 Weeks)		**9,082**	**9,005**	**4,277**	**4,277**	**1,503**	**1,493**	**5,530**	**766**	**25,907**

≠ The weekly deaths are compiled on receipt of death registration documents prior to coding or checking and are therefore provisional.
**Including bronchiolitis.
††Except secondary to accidents and to other infections (including influenza).

Table 3 Notification rates per 100,000 population for selected infectious diseases: sex and age-group, 1990

England and Wales

Age-group	Food poisoning									Malaria		
	All			Formally notified			Ascertained by other means					
	P	M	F	P	M	F	P	M	F	P	M	F
All ages ψ	**103**	**106**	**100**	**73**	**75**	**70**	**30**	**31**	**29**	**3**	**4**	**2**
0 - 4	234	244	222	163	171	154	71	74	68	2	2	*1*
5 - 14	73	80	66	51	56	46	22	24	20	3	3	2
15 - 24	113	112	115	83	83	82	31	29	32	4	5	3
25 - 44	112	113	111	82	82	81	30	30	30	4	5	3
45 - 64	73	72	75	53	52	54	20	20	21	2	3	2
65 and over	54	55	54	39	39	38	15	15	16	1	1	*0**

Age-group	Scarlet fever			Age-group	Meningitis						Meningococcal septicaemia (without meningitis)		
					All			Meningococcal					
	P	M	F		P	M	F	P	M	F	P	M	F
All ages ψ	**14**	**14**	**14**	All ages ψ	**5**	**5**	**5**	**2**	**2**	**2**	**1**	**1**	**1**
0	15	14	16	0	88	93	83	36	38	33	9	10	8
1	40	40	39	1	51	56	46	21	22	19	6	6	7
2	67	71	63	2	26	27	25	12	13	11	4	5	*3*
3	119	117	121	3	19	21	17	8	8	9	2	2	2
4	157	162	152	4	11	12	10	5	7	*3*	2	2	2
5	161	156	167	5 - 9	6	7	5	3	4	3	1	*1*	*1*
6	111	100	123	10 - 14	5	5	5	2	2	3	*1*	*1*	*1*
7	70	55	86	15 - 24	5	5	4	3	3	3	*0**	*1*	*0**
8	52	44	61	25 and over	1	1	2	*0**	*0**	1	*0**	*0**	*0**
9	43	34	52										
10 - 14	20	18	21										
15 - 24	8	9	7										
25 - 44	3	2	3										
45 and over	*0**	*0**	*0**										

Age-group	Tuberculosis ≠ (excluding chemoprophylaxis)											
	All			Respiratory †			Meningitis †			Other forms †		
	P	M	F	P	M	F	P	M	F	P	M	F
All ages ψ	**10**	**12**	**9**	**8**	**9**	**6**	**0***	**0***	**0***	**2**	**2**	**3**
0	*2*	*2*	*2*	*1*	*1*	*1*	-	-	-	*1*	*0**	*1*
1	4	*4*	5	*3*	*3*	*3*	*0**	*0**	-	*1*	*1*	*2*
2 - 4	5	5	6	3	3	4	*0**	*0**	*0**	2	2	2
5 - 9	4	4	4	3	3	3	*0**	*0**	-	1	1	*1*
10 - 14	4	4	4	3	3	3	*0**	-	*0**	1	*1*	*2*
15 - 19	6	5	6	4	4	4	*0**	*0**	*0**	1	1	2
20 - 24	11	10	11	7	7	8	*0**	*0**	*0**	3	3	3
25 - 34	11	11	12	8	8	8	*0**	*0**	*0**	3	3	4
35 - 44	10	11	9	7	8	6	*0**	*0**	*0**	3	3	3
45 - 54	11	12	10	8	10	6	*0**	*0**	*0**	3	2	3
55 - 64	14	16	11	10	13	8	*0**	*0**	*0**	3	3	3
65 - 74	14	21	9	12	18	7	*0**	*0**	*0**	2	2	2
75 and over	16	27	11	14	24	8	*0**	*0**	*0**	2	3	2

ψ Includes age unknown.
* Less than 0.5.
† Categories overlap and therefore some cases will be included in more than one column.
≠ See note on page vi.

Table 3 Series MB2 no.17

Table 3 - *continued*

Age-group	Dysentery		
	P	M	F
All agesψ	**5**	**5**	**6**
0	12	13	11
1	21	22	19
2	18	20	16
3	18	21	16
4	15	14	16
5 - 9	11	11	11
10 - 14	5	5	5
15 - 24	5	4	6
25 - 64	4	4	5
65 and over	1	1	1

Age-group	Viral hepatitis		
	P	M	F
All agesψ	**18**	**19**	**16**
0	2	3	2
1	5	7	3
2 - 4	21	21	21
5 - 9	57	55	59
10 - 14	42	43	42
15 - 19	25	27	22
20 - 24	23	25	21
25 - 34	23	24	22
35 - 44	13	14	12
45 - 54	7	8	6
55 - 64	4	4	4
65 - 74	2	3	2
75 and over	2	2	1

Age-group	Whooping cough		
	P	M	F
All agesψ	**30**	**29**	**32**
Under 3 months**	222	197	248
3 - 5 months**	326	329	323
6 - 8 months**	212	204	221
9 - 11 months**	169	153	185
1	175	167	183
2	232	206	260
3	255	227	284
4	255	237	274
5	271	242	303
6	256	231	283
7	163	140	186
8	105	94	116
9	89	72	107
10 - 14	33	31	36
15 - 19	4	4	5
20 - 24	2	2	2
25 - 34	2	2	3
35 - 44	2	2	3
45 - 54	1	1	1
55 - 64	1	1	1
65 - 74	0*	0*	1
75 and over	0*	0*	0*

Age-group	Measles		
	P	M	F
All agesψ	**26**	**28**	**24**
Under 1 month††	63	68	57
1 month††	77	65	90
2 months††	135	144	126
3 months††	165	174	154
4 months††	250	280	219
5 months††	343	304	384
6 months††	590	625	552
7 months††	576	537	617
8 months††	737	718	757
9 months††	753	755	750
10 months††	760	793	725
11 months††	751	745	757
1	408	404	412
2	166	170	163
3	125	129	121
4	125	132	119
5	109	113	105
6	97	91	103
7	79	80	77
8	60	61	59
9	54	51	58
10 - 14	27	31	24
15 - 24	10	13	6
25 and over	1	1	1

Age-group	Rubella			Mumps		
	P	M	F	P	M	F
All agesψ	**23**	**25**	**20**	**8**	**9**	**8**
0	265	266	263	11	14	9
1	234	236	232	43	56	29
2	108	108	107	43	48	37
3	110	117	103	62	78	47
4	124	132	116	81	91	72
5	113	118	108	59	66	52
6	116	112	120	53	54	52
7	96	85	108	40	45	35
8	84	75	94	33	35	32
9	74	76	72	27	26	28
10 - 14	30	35	24	15	14	15
15 - 24	15	23	6	4	3	5
25 and over	2	2	1	2	2	2

ψ   Includes age unknown.
*   Less than 0.5.
**   Calculated using a quarter of the population at risk under 1 year.
††   Calculated using a twelfth of the population at risk under 1 year.

Table 4 Series MB2 no.17

**Table 4 Notifications of selected infectious diseases:
sex and age-group, 1990**

Final numbers after correction

Age-group	Sex	England and Wales (excluding port health authorities)	Wales	North	Yorkshire and Humberside	East Midlands	East Anglia	South East	South West	West Midlands	North West
Typhoid Fever contracted abroad											
All ages	**M**	**73**	**-**	**-**	**17**	**8**	**-**	**33**	**2**	**8**	**5**
	F	**50**	**1**	**1**	**8**	**2**	**-**	**29**	**-**	**4**	**5**
0 - 4 years	M	7	-	-	-	-	-	6	-	1	-
	F	6	-	-	3	-	-	2	-	1	-
5 - 14 years	M	13	-	-	2	3	-	5	1	1	1
	F	14	1	1	1	-	-	10	-	-	1
15 - 24 years	M	19	-	-	6	1	-	11	1	-	-
	F	12	-	-	2	1	-	5	-	2	2
25 - 44 years	M	21	-	-	4	2	-	8	-	4	3
	F	14	-	-	1	1	-	9	-	1	2
45 - 64 years	M	8	-	-	3	2	-	-	-	2	1
	F	3	-	-	1	-	-	2	-	-	-
65 - and over	M	-	-	-	-	-	-	-	-	-	-
	F	-	-	-	-	-	-	-	-	-	-
Unknown	M	5	-	-	2	-	-	3	-	-	-
	F	1	-	-	-	-	-	1	-	-	-
Typhoid Fever contracted in Great Britain											
All ages	**M**	**13**	**-**	**1**	**3**	**-**	**1**	**5**	**-**	**1**	**2**
	F	**9**	**-**	**-**	**-**	**-**	**-**	**8**	**-**	**-**	**1**
0 - 4 years	M	3	-	-	-	-	1	2	-	-	-
	F	1	-	-	-	-	-	1	-	-	-
5 - 14 years	M	1	-	-	1	-	-	-	-	-	-
	F	5	-	-	-	-	-	5	-	-	-
15 - 24 years	M	3	-	-	1	-	-	-	-	1	1
	F	-	-	-	-	-	-	-	-	-	-
25 - 44 years	M	3	-	-	-	-	-	2	-	-	1
	F	3	-	-	-	-	-	2	-	-	1
45 - 64 years	M	1	-	-	1	-	-	-	-	-	-
	F	-	-	-	-	-	-	-	-	-	-
65 - and over	M	1	-	-	-	-	-	1	-	-	-
	F	-	-	-	-	-	-	-	-	-	-
Unknown	M	1	-	1	-	-	-	-	-	-	-
	F	-	-	-	-	-	-	-	-	-	-
Typhoid Fever contracted ns											
All ages	**M**	**23**	**-**	**-**	**1**	**-**	**-**	**14**	**-**	**6**	**2**
	F	**9**	**-**	**-**	**-**	**-**	**-**	**4**	**-**	**4**	**1**
0 - 4 years	M	-	-	-	-	-	-	-	-	-	-
	F	1	-	-	-	-	-	1	-	-	-
5 - 14 years	M	7	-	-	-	-	-	5	-	2	-
	F	1	-	-	-	-	-	-	-	-	1
15 - 24 years	M	7	-	-	-	-	-	4	-	2	1
	F	1	-	-	-	-	-	-	-	1	-
25 - 44 years	M	4	-	-	1	-	-	3	-	-	-
	F	3	-	-	-	-	-	2	-	1	-
45 - 64 years	M	3	-	-	-	-	-	1	-	2	-
	F	1	-	-	-	-	-	-	-	1	-
65 - and over	M	-	-	-	-	-	-	-	-	-	-
	F	-	-	-	-	-	-	-	-	-	-
Unknown	M	2	-	-	-	-	-	1	-	-	1
	F	2	-	-	-	-	-	1	-	1	-

See note on page viii.

**England and Wales,
standard regions,
regional health authorities**

Regional health authorities

North-ern	York-shire	Trent	East Anglian	North West Thames	North East Thames	South East Thames	South West Thames	Wessex	Oxford	South West-ern	West Mid-lands	Mersey	North West-ern	Sex	Age-group
Typhoid Fever contracted abroad															
-	**14**	**9**	-	**14**	**7**	**4**	**4**	-	**6**	**2**	**8**	**1**	**4**	M	All ages
1	**6**	**4**	-	**15**	**5**	**3**	**5**	-	**1**	-	**4**	-	**5**	F	
-	-	-	-	2	2	1	1	-	-	-	1	-	-	M	0 - 4 years
-	3	-	-	-	2	-	-	-	-	-	1	-	-	F	
-	2	3	-	3	-	-	-	-	2	1	1	-	1	M	5 - 14 years
1	-	1	-	5	2	-	3	-	-	-	-	-	1	F	
-	5	2	-	4	3	1	2	-	1	1	-	-	-	M	15 - 24 years
-	2	1	-	2	1	1	1	-	-	-	2	-	2	F	
-	3	3	-	4	2	1	1	-	-	-	4	1	2	M	25 - 44 years
-	-	2	-	5	-	2	1	-	1	-	1	-	2	F	
-	2	1	-	-	-	-	-	-	2	-	2	-	1	M	45 - 64 years
-	1	-	-	2	-	-	-	-	-	-	-	-	-	F	
-	-	-	-	-	-	-	-	-	-	-	-	-	-	M	65 and over
-	-	-	-	-	-	-	-	-	-	-	-	-	-	F	
-	2	-	-	1	-	1	-	-	1	-	-	-	-	M	Unknown
-	-	-	-	1	-	-	-	-	-	-	-	-	-	F	
Typhoid Fever contracted in Great Britain															
1	**3**	-	**1**	**1**	**3**	**1**	-	-	-	-	**1**	-	**2**	M	All ages
-	-	-	-	**6**	**1**	-	**1**	-	-	-	-	-	**1**	F	
-	-	-	1	1	-	1	-	-	-	-	-	-	-	M	0 - 4 years
-	-	-	-	-	-	1	-	-	-	-	-	-	-	F	
-	1	-	-	-	-	-	-	-	-	-	-	-	-	M	5 - 14 years
-	-	-	-	5	-	-	-	-	-	-	-	-	-	F	
-	1	-	-	-	-	-	-	-	-	-	1	-	1	M	15 - 24 years
-	-	-	-	-	-	-	-	-	-	-	-	-	-	F	
-	-	-	-	-	2	-	-	-	-	-	-	-	1	M	25 - 44 years
-	-	-	-	1	1	-	-	-	-	-	-	-	1	F	
-	1	-	-	-	-	-	-	-	-	-	-	-	-	M	45 - 64 years
-	-	-	-	-	-	-	-	-	-	-	-	-	-	F	
-	-	-	-	-	1	-	-	-	-	-	-	-	-	M	65 and over
-	-	-	-	-	-	-	-	-	-	-	-	-	-	F	
1	-	-	-	-	-	-	-	-	-	-	-	-	-	M	Unknown
-	-	-	-	-	-	-	-	-	-	-	-	-	-	F	
Typhoid Fever contracted ns															
-	**1**	-	-	**2**	**7**	**2**	**2**	-	**1**	-	**6**	-	**2**	M	All ages
-	-	-	-	**2**	**2**	-	-	-	-	-	**4**	-	**1**	F	
-	-	-	-	-	-	-	-	-	-	-	-	-	-	M	0 - 4 years
-	-	-	-	-	1	-	-	-	-	-	-	-	-	F	
-	-	-	-	-	3	1	1	-	-	-	2	-	-	M	5 - 14 years
-	-	-	-	-	-	-	-	-	-	-	-	-	1	F	
-	-	-	-	1	1	1	-	-	1	-	2	-	1	M	15 - 24 years
-	-	-	-	-	-	-	-	-	-	-	1	-	-	F	
-	1	-	-	1	2	-	-	-	-	-	1	-	-	M	25 - 44 years
-	-	-	-	1	1	-	-	-	-	-	1	-	-	F	
-	-	-	-	-	-	-	1	-	-	-	2	-	-	M	45 - 64 years
-	-	-	-	-	-	-	-	-	-	-	1	-	-	F	
-	-	-	-	-	-	-	-	-	-	-	-	-	-	M	65 and over
-	-	-	-	-	-	-	-	-	-	-	-	-	-	F	
-	-	-	-	-	1	-	-	-	-	-	-	-	1	M	Unknown
-	-	-	-	1	-	-	-	-	-	-	1	-	-	F	

Table 4 Series MB2 no.17

Table 4 - *continued*

Age-group	Sex	England and Wales (excluding port health authorities)	Wales	Standard regions							
				North	Yorkshire and Humberside	East Midlands	East Anglia	South East	South West	West Midlands	North West
Paratyphoid Fever contracted abroad											
All ages	**M**	**41**	-	-	**4**	**3**	**2**	**14**	**1**	**12**	**5**
	F	**23**	-	-	**4**	**1**	-	**12**	**1**	**2**	**3**
0 - 4 years	M	1	-	-	-	-	-	1	-	-	-
	F	-	-	-	-	-	-	-	-	-	-
5 - 14 years	M	5	-	-	1	-	-	3	-	1	-
	F	2	-	-	-	-	-	2	-	-	-
15 - 24 years	M	9	-	-	-	-	1	-	-	4	4
	F	5	-	-	1	-	-	1	-	-	3
25 - 44 years	M	19	-	-	2	2	-	6	1	7	1
	F	13	-	-	3	1	-	7	-	2	-
45 - 64 years	M	5	-	-	1	1	-	3	-	-	-
	F	2	-	-	-	-	-	1	1	-	-
65 - and over	M	-	-	-	-	-	-	-	-	-	-
	F	-	-	-	-	-	-	-	-	-	-
Unknown	M	2	-	-	-	-	1	1	-	-	-
	F	1	-	-	-	-	-	1	-	-	-
Paratyphoid Fever contracted in Great Britain											
All ages	**M**	**11**	-	-	**2**	-	**1**	**3**	-	**1**	**4**
	F	**2**	1	-	-	-	-	-	-	-	1
0 - 4 years	M	2	-	-	-	-	1	1	-	-	-
	F	-	-	-	-	-	-	-	-	-	-
5 - 14 years	M	2	-	-	-	-	-	-	-	1	1
	F	-	-	-	-	-	-	-	-	-	-
15 - 24 years	M	1	-	-	-	-	-	1	-	-	-
	F	-	-	-	-	-	-	-	-	-	-
25 - 44 years	M	3	-	-	-	-	-	-	-	-	3
	F	-	-	-	-	-	-	-	-	-	-
45 - 64 years	M	-	-	-	-	-	-	-	-	-	-
	F	1	1	-	-	-	-	-	-	-	-
65 - and over	M	2	-	-	2	-	-	-	-	-	-
	F	1	-	-	-	-	-	-	-	-	1
Unknown	M	1	-	-	-	-	-	1	-	-	-
	F	-	-	-	-	-	-	-	-	-	-
Paratyphoid Fever contracted ns											
All ages	**M**	**9**	-	**2**	-	-	-	**4**	**2**	-	**1**
	F	**7**	-	**1**	**3**	-	-	**2**	-	**1**	-
0 - 4 years	M	-	-	-	-	-	-	-	-	-	-
	F	-	-	-	-	-	-	-	-	-	-
5 - 14 years	M	-	-	-	-	-	-	-	-	-	-
	F	1	-	-	-	-	-	1	-	-	-
15 - 24 years	M	4	-	-	-	-	-	4	-	-	-
	F	1	-	-	1	-	-	-	-	-	-
25 - 44 years	M	3	-	1	-	-	-	-	1	-	1
	F	4	-	1	1	-	-	1	-	1	-
45 - 64 years	M	1	-	1	-	-	-	-	-	-	-
	F	1	-	-	1	-	-	-	-	-	-
65 - and over	M	-	-	-	-	-	-	-	-	-	-
	F	-	-	-	-	-	-	-	-	-	-
Unknown	M	1	-	-	-	-	-	-	1	-	-
	F	-	-	-	-	-	-	-	-	-	-

Regional health authorities														Sex	Age-group
North-ern	York-shire	Trent	East Anglian	North West Thames	North East Thames	South East Thames	South West Thames	Wessex	Oxford	South West-ern	West Mid-lands	Mersey	North West-ern		
Paratyphoid Fever contracted abroad															
-	4	3	2	6	5	-	1	-	2	1	12	1	4	M	All ages
-	4	1	-	6	2	1	3	-	-	1	2	-	3	F	
-	-	-	-	1	-	-	-	-	-	-	-	-	-	M	0 - 4 years
-	-	-	-	-	-	-	-	-	-	-	-	-	-	F	
-	1	-	-	-	2	-	-	-	1	-	1	-	-	M	5 - 14 years
-	-	-	-	1	-	-	1	-	-	-	-	-	-	F	
-	-	-	1	-	-	-	-	-	-	-	4	1	3	M	15 - 24 years
-	1	-	-	-	1	-	-	-	-	-	-	-	3	F	
-	2	2	-	4	2	-	-	-	-	1	7	-	1	M	25 - 44 years
-	3	1	-	4	1	1	1	-	-	-	2	-	-	F	
-	1	1	-	-	1	-	1	-	1	-	-	-	-	M	45 - 64 years
-	-	-	-	1	-	-	-	-	-	1	-	-	-	F	
-	-	-	-	-	-	-	-	-	-	-	-	-	-	M	65 and over
-	-	-	-	-	-	-	-	-	-	-	-	-	-	F	
-	-	-	1	1	-	-	-	-	-	-	-	-	-	M	Unknown
-	-	-	-	-	-	-	1	-	-	-	-	-	-	F	
Paratyphoid Fever contracted in Great Britain															
-	2	-	1	1	2	-	-	-	-	-	1	1	3	M	All ages
-	-	-	-	-	-	-	-	-	-	-	-	-	1	F	
-	-	-	1	-	1	-	-	-	-	-	-	-	-	M	0 - 4 years
-	-	-	-	-	-	-	-	-	-	-	-	-	-	F	
-	-	-	-	-	-	-	-	-	-	-	1	-	1	M	5 - 14 years
-	-	-	-	-	-	-	-	-	-	-	-	-	-	F	
-	-	-	-	1	-	-	-	-	-	-	-	-	-	M	15 - 24 years
-	-	-	-	-	-	-	-	-	-	-	-	-	-	F	
-	-	-	-	-	-	-	-	-	-	-	-	1	2	M	25 - 44 years
-	-	-	-	-	-	-	-	-	-	-	-	-	-	F	
-	-	-	-	-	-	-	-	-	-	-	-	-	-	M	45 - 64 years
-	-	-	-	-	-	-	-	-	-	-	-	-	-	F	
-	2	-	-	-	-	-	-	-	-	-	-	-	-	M	65 and over
-	-	-	-	-	-	-	-	-	-	-	-	-	1	F	
-	-	-	-	-	1	-	-	-	-	-	-	-	-	M	Unknown
-	-	-	-	-	-	-	-	-	-	-	-	-	-	F	
Paratyphoid Fever contracted ns															
2	-	-	-	-	3	-	-	1	1	1	-	-	1	M	All ages
1	3	-	-	-	-	1	-	-	1	-	1	-	-	F	
-	-	-	-	-	-	-	-	-	-	-	-	-	-	M	0 - 4 years
-	-	-	-	-	-	-	-	-	-	-	-	-	-	F	
-	-	-	-	-	-	-	-	-	-	-	-	-	-	M	5 - 14 years
-	-	-	-	-	-	-	-	1	-	-	-	-	-	F	
-	-	-	-	-	3	-	-	-	1	-	-	-	-	M	15 - 24 years
-	1	-	-	-	-	-	-	-	-	-	-	-	-	F	
1	-	-	-	-	-	-	-	1	-	-	-	-	1	M	25 - 44 years
1	1	-	-	-	-	1	-	-	-	-	1	-	-	F	
1	-	-	-	-	-	-	-	-	-	-	-	-	-	M	45 - 64 years
-	1	-	-	-	-	-	-	-	-	-	-	-	-	F	
-	-	-	-	-	-	-	-	-	-	-	-	-	-	M	65 and over
-	-	-	-	-	-	-	-	-	-	-	-	-	-	F	
-	-	-	-	-	-	-	-	-	-	1	-	-	-	M	Unknown
-	-	-	-	-	-	-	-	-	-	-	-	-	-	F	

Table 4 Series MB2 no.17

Table 4 - *continued*

Age-group	Sex	England and Wales (excluding port health authorities)	Wales	Standard regions							
				North	Yorkshire and Humberside	East Midlands	East Anglia	South East	South West	West Midlands	North West
Food poisoning, formally notified											
All ages	M	**18,688**	**1,279**	**1,462**	**2,500**	**1,562**	**588**	**6,372**	**1,661**	**1,419**	**1,845**
	F	**18,257**	**1,249**	**1,419**	**2,502**	**1,569**	**576**	**5,948**	**1,621**	**1,412**	**1,961**
0 - 4 years	M	2,953	221	241	436	207	81	932	267	228	340
	F	2,545	185	207	353	194	64	842	201	177	322
5 - 14 years	M	1,787	147	154	251	103	48	589	182	128	185
	F	1,396	126	104	187	96	52	473	123	90	145
15 - 24 years	M	3,151	206	211	454	277	101	1,100	271	249	282
	F	2,990	195	212	412	250	96	1,051	276	227	271
25 - 44 years	M	6,120	396	456	764	562	195	2,250	515	447	535
	F	5,925	397	439	797	544	183	2,027	505	438	595
45 - 64 years	M	2,828	184	234	355	261	88	953	265	225	263
	F	2,955	203	231	374	283	100	923	275	248	318
65 and over	M	1,274	82	118	185	102	50	355	138	86	158
	F	1,848	85	157	329	155	65	483	219	141	214
Unknown	M	575	43	48	55	50	25	193	23	56	82
	F	598	58	69	50	47	16	149	22	91	96
Food poisoning, ascertained by other means											
All ages	M	**7,577**	**227**	**536**	**1,043**	**465**	**120**	**2,132**	**904**	**1,222**	**928**
	F	**7,623**	**268**	**511**	**1,123**	**441**	**134**	**2,028**	**938**	**1,326**	**854**
0 - 4 years	M	1,277	22	86	209	90	18	320	129	215	188
	F	1,124	20	78	197	65	14	276	136	186	152
5 - 14 years	M	752	20	63	106	48	5	218	87	118	87
	F	589	18	36	75	35	8	186	67	102	62
15 - 24 years	M	1,098	42	68	147	78	18	312	131	194	108
	F	1,173	46	64	150	78	21	339	145	223	107
25 - 44 years	M	2,259	71	154	277	129	45	664	266	410	243
	F	2,233	90	163	291	124	47	602	282	406	228
45 - 64 years	M	1,080	35	93	118	58	18	297	183	160	118
	F	1,149	53	78	152	59	20	267	184	220	116
65 and over	M	493	18	42	92	30	7	117	71	77	39
	F	745	28	57	122	48	22	162	85	146	75
Unknown	M	618	19	30	94	32	9	204	37	48	145
	F	610	13	35	136	32	2	196	39	43	114
Dysentery											
All ages	M	**1,303**	**101**	**25**	**252**	**68**	**23**	**475**	**102**	**110**	**147**
	F	**1,453**	**134**	**23**	**300**	**59**	**24**	**520**	**146**	**88**	**159**
Under 1 year	M	47	4	-	16	3	-	11	3	3	7
	F	37	5	1	12	1	-	7	2	1	8
1 year	M	76	6	-	19	4	-	22	5	5	15
	F	64	7	1	20	4	-	15	6	4	7
2 years	M	71	6	1	21	1	-	22	4	8	8
	F	53	4	-	8	1	-	18	7	4	11
3 years	M	71	4	-	14	6	1	17	9	9	11
	F	51	12	1	9	4	-	9	6	3	7
4 years	M	48	4	1	18	3	-	8	4	2	8
	F	53	7	1	12	2	-	13	5	3	10
5 - 9 years	M	177	25	3	32	13	1	51	13	16	23
	F	166	32	3	41	6	-	31	19	10	24
10 - 14 years	M	77	8	2	22	5	-	18	2	12	8
	F	68	13	1	11	2	-	19	8	6	8
15 - 24 years	M	162	5	3	21	9	7	76	16	13	12
	F	206	12	4	44	4	8	87	22	9	16
25 - 64 years	M	512	30	15	81	24	13	235	44	30	40
	F	642	34	9	111	30	14	293	59	42	50
65 and over	M	24	1	-	5	-	1	7	-	8	2
	F	67	2	1	24	4	-	14	7	5	10
Unknown	M	38	8	-	3	-	-	8	2	4	13
	F	46	6	1	8	1	2	14	5	1	8

North ern	York- shire	Trent	East Anglian	North West Thames	North East Thames	South East Thames	South West Thames	Wessex	Oxford	South West- ern	West Mid- lands	Mersey	North West- ern	Sex	Age-group
Regional health authorities														**Sex**	**Age-group**

Food poisoning, formally notified

North ern	York- shire	Trent	East Anglian	North West Thames	North East Thames	South East Thames	South West Thames	Wessex	Oxford	South West- ern	West Mid- lands	Mersey	North West- ern	Sex	Age-group
1,462	**1,948**	**1,807**	**588**	**1,305**	**1,410**	**1,308**	**1,113**	**747**	**1,168**	**1,289**	**1,419**	**802**	**1,043**	**M**	All ages
1,419	**1,972**	**1,814**	**576**	**1,202**	**1,346**	**1,194**	**1,047**	**821**	**1,023**	**1,221**	**1,412**	**868**	**1,093**	**F**	
241	338	254	81	202	217	184	168	114	168	197	228	129	211	M	0 - 4 years
207	294	215	64	178	196	154	151	112	145	145	177	136	186	F	
154	209	113	48	130	128	134	82	70	104	155	128	75	110	M	5 - 14 years
104	158	107	52	101	114	111	66	57	67	98	90	68	77	F	
211	342	344	101	213	258	210	194	141	195	205	249	141	141	M	15 - 24 years
212	316	298	96	206	261	203	176	149	178	202	227	129	142	F	
456	607	601	195	469	469	455	404	223	454	409	447	268	267	M	25 - 44 years
439	616	631	183	412	438	397	380	259	369	371	438	273	322	F	
234	259	315	88	187	195	206	171	121	179	201	225	111	152	M	45 - 64 years
231	296	297	100	179	180	197	159	153	182	212	248	146	172	F	
118	140	130	50	67	84	83	54	64	53	105	86	64	94	M	65 and over
157	250	213	65	91	111	108	87	84	66	176	141	88	126	F	
48	53	50	25	37	59	36	40	14	15	17	56	14	68	M	Unknown
69	42	53	16	35	46	24	28	7	16	17	91	28	68	F	

Food poisoning, ascertained by other means

North ern	York- shire	Trent	East Anglian	North West Thames	North East Thames	South East Thames	South West Thames	Wessex	Oxford	South West- ern	West Mid- lands	Mersey	North West- ern	Sex	Age-group
536	**838**	**617**	**120**	**375**	**398**	**395**	**474**	**562**	**257**	**628**	**1,222**	**61**	**867**	**M**	All ages
511	**883**	**630**	**134**	**356**	**377**	**385**	**439**	**585**	**231**	**644**	**1,326**	**82**	**772**	**F**	
86	178	111	18	54	61	56	67	78	40	103	215	12	176	M	0 - 4 years
78	167	88	14	37	56	62	61	58	41	104	186	11	141	F	
63	85	65	5	52	43	48	38	35	23	70	118	4	83	M	5 - 14 years
36	58	47	8	36	31	37	38	40	27	49	102	7	55	F	
68	117	99	18	43	69	69	68	72	39	92	194	9	99	M	15 - 24 years
64	126	92	21	64	62	64	67	101	37	99	223	13	94	F	
154	227	160	45	108	128	130	147	161	94	181	410	19	224	M	25 - 44 years
163	247	152	47	117	123	109	126	169	65	191	406	24	204	F	
93	97	72	18	48	52	54	70	117	44	102	160	7	111	M	45 - 64 years
78	121	82	20	29	51	65	67	103	33	111	220	9	107	F	
42	74	46	7	18	27	19	27	45	11	43	77	3	36	M	65 and over
57	97	69	22	23	33	29	39	55	20	52	146	10	65	F	
30	60	64	9	52	18	19	57	54	6	37	48	7	138	M	Unknown
35	67	100	2	50	21	19	41	59	8	38	43	8	106	F	

Dysentery

North ern	York- shire	Trent	East Anglian	North West Thames	North East Thames	South East Thames	South West Thames	Wessex	Oxford	South West- ern	West Mid- lands	Mersey	North West- ern	Sex	Age-group
25	**236**	**76**	**23**	**152**	**96**	**71**	**73**	**33**	**80**	**80**	**110**	**20**	**127**	**M**	All ages
23	**283**	**69**	**24**	**145**	**113**	**60**	**104**	**52**	**91**	**108**	**88**	**15**	**144**	**F**	
-	15	4	-	1	3	-	6	-	1	3	3	2	5	M	Under 1 year
1	12	1	-	3	1	1	1	1	1	1	1	-	8	F	
-	18	5	-	9	4	5	2	1	2	4	5	2	13	M	1 year
1	18	6	-	5	4	-	3	1	3	5	4	-	7	F	
1	21	1	-	6	5	6	3	-	2	4	8	-	8	M	2 years
-	7	1	-	5	6	2	3	-	3	7	4	-	11	F	
-	10	10	1	6	3	5	2	1	1	8	9	-	11	M	3 years
1	8	5	-	1	3	1	2	1	2	5	3	-	7	F	
1	18	3	-	5	2	1	-	2	-	2	2	2	6	M	4 years
1	12	2	-	7	2	1	2	-	1	5	3	-	10	F	
3	31	13	1	21	12	8	3	2	7	12	16	2	21	M	5 - 9 years
3	41	6	-	14	9	1	5	3	2	16	10	3	21	F	
2	20	7	-	4	5	3	-	1	6	1	12	1	7	M	10 - 14 years
1	10	3	-	7	4	2	3	5	2	4	6	-	8	F	
3	19	9	7	12	18	14	17	8	13	12	13	-	12	M	15 - 24 years
4	40	8	8	18	18	6	17	10	22	18	9	1	15	F	
15	76	24	13	83	42	27	39	16	43	34	30	10	30	M	25 - 64 years
9	106	31	14	77	60	41	63	24	51	40	42	8	42	F	
-	5	-	1	2	-	2	-	-	3	-	8	1	1	M	65 and over
1	22	4	-	4	3	4	1	5	3	3	5	3	7	F	
-	3	-	-	3	2	-	1	2	2	-	4	-	13	M	Unknown
1	7	2	2	4	3	1	4	2	1	4	1	-	8	F	

Table 4 Series MB2 no.17

Table 4 - *continued*

Age-group	Sex	England and Wales (excluding port health authorities)	Wales	Standard regions							
				North	Yorkshire and Humberside	East Midlands	East Anglia	South East	South West	West Midlands	North West
All tuberculosis*											
All ages	M	**2,865**	**123**	**123**	**304**	**214**	**51**	**1,162**	**105**	**383**	**400**
	F	**2,339**	**71**	**82**	**233**	**190**	**46**	**957**	**68**	**349**	**343**
Under 1 year	M	6	-	-	-	-	-	3	-	1	2
	F	6	-	-	-	1	1	1	-	2	1
1 year	M	14	-	-	2	-	1	7	-	3	1
	F	16	2	-	1	1	2	3	1	3	3
2 - 4 years	M	53	1	1	7	3	-	18	-	8	15
	F	56	3	1	12	4	1	12	1	7	15
5 - 9 years	M	64	2	1	8	5	1	20	2	10	15
	F	60	3	3	5	2	1	24	1	6	15
10 - 14 years	M	59	2	3	7	1	-	20	-	13	13
	F	65	1	2	7	7	1	22	-	13	12
15 - 19 years	M	94	2	-	13	8	3	35	3	20	10
	F	101	-	2	11	10	2	31	-	23	22
20 - 24 years	M	197	4	-	21	15	2	94	3	34	24
	F	224	3	5	26	27	3	91	5	32	32
25 - 34 years	M	431	14	17	32	30	3	232	11	43	49
	F	449	6	10	36	37	5	242	11	48	54
35 - 44 years	M	373	12	13	42	30	10	166	11	43	46
	F	302	3	3	35	27	6	138	6	41	43
45 - 54 years	M	351	16	17	36	19	6	144	14	52	47
	F	278	8	13	26	15	3	120	4	58	31
55 - 64 years	M	414	20	21	44	33	10	162	9	52	63
	F	284	7	18	27	19	8	105	12	45	43
65 - 74 years	M	413	23	25	46	43	8	139	27	49	53
	F	212	17	6	25	23	6	66	11	29	29
75 and over	M	326	27	23	40	24	7	94	24	43	44
	F	248	17	18	20	15	6	85	15	37	35
Unknown	M	70	-	2	6	3	-	28	1	12	18
	F	38	1	1	2	2	1	17	1	5	8
Tuberculosis, respiratory†											
All ages	M	**2,295**	**109**	**105**	**236**	**178**	**42**	**911**	**95**	**289**	**330**
	F	**1,647**	**54**	**65**	**162**	**153**	**31**	**678**	**45**	**222**	**237**
Under 1 year	M	5	-	-	-	-	-	3	-	1	1
	F	2	-	-	-	1	-	-	-	1	-
1 year	M	10	-	-	2	-	-	5	-	2	1
	F	9	1	-	-	-	1	2	1	1	3
2 - 4 years	M	29	-	1	2	1	-	11	-	4	10
	F	39	2	-	7	4	-	9	-	5	12
5 - 9 years	M	42	1	1	7	5	-	10	1	7	10
	F	42	2	2	3	2	1	17	-	3	12
10 - 14 years	M	42	1	3	6	-	-	12	-	9	11
	F	40	1	2	3	5	1	16	-	7	5
15 - 19 years	M	72	2	-	10	5	3	28	2	14	8
	F	72	-	2	7	5	1	21	-	17	19
20 - 24 years	M	145	4	-	12	14	2	68	3	24	18
	F	155	3	3	20	22	3	61	3	22	18
25 - 34 years	M	331	11	13	21	25	3	181	9	29	39
	F	315	5	8	26	30	4	169	8	31	34
35 - 44 years	M	277	10	11	29	26	6	119	11	30	35
	F	196	2	2	24	20	4	89	6	22	27
45 - 54 years	M	285	14	14	28	14	6	118	14	37	40
	F	184	5	10	16	14	3	83	2	33	18
55 - 64 years	M	336	19	16	37	25	8	132	7	38	54
	F	203	6	15	16	18	5	75	6	31	31
65 - 74 years	M	369	20	22	42	36	7	123	27	44	48
	F	167	13	5	21	19	4	53	7	22	23
75 and over	M	293	27	22	34	24	7	78	20	42	39
	F	192	13	15	17	11	4	69	11	24	28
Unknown	M	59	-	2	6	3	-	23	1	8	16
	F	31	1	1	2	2	-	14	1	3	7

* Excludes chemoprophylaxis, see note on page vi.
† Specificity codes 23.1, .2, .5, .6, .7, .8.

Regional health authorities														Sex	Age-group
North-ern	York-shire	Trent	East Anglian	North West Thames	North East Thames	South East Thames	South West Thames	Wessex	Oxford	South West-ern	West Mid-lands	Mersey	North West-ern		
All tuberculosis*															
123	**246**	**245**	**51**	**351**	**370**	**221**	**132**	**69**	**85**	**66**	**383**	**75**	**325**	M	All ages
82	**191**	**207**	**46**	**294**	**300**	**161**	**126**	**42**	**79**	**48**	**349**	**64**	**279**	F	
-	-	-	-	-	-	3	-	-	-	-	1	-	2	M	Under 1 year
-	-	-	1	-	-	1	-	-	1	-	2	-	1	F	
-	2	-	1	1	2	3	1	-	-	-	3	-	1	M	1 year
-	1	1	2	1	2	-	-	-	-	1	3	-	3	F	
1	6	3	-	3	5	5	2	1	3	-	8	2	13	M	2 - 4 years
1	8	8	1	3	3	2	1	2	1	1	7	3	12	F	
1	8	5	1	3	10	5	1	-	1	2	10	2	13	M	5 - 9 years
3	3	2	1	5	8	6	2	2	3	1	6	1	14	F	
3	5	3	-	4	6	5	1	3	1	-	13	-	13	M	10 - 14 years
2	6	7	1	9	8	4	-	1	1	-	13	-	12	F	
-	10	10	3	6	15	9	4	2	1	2	20	1	9	M	15 - 19 years
2	10	10	2	9	10	7	3	1	2	-	23	4	18	F	
-	19	16	2	36	37	6	5	4	9	1	34	5	19	M	20 - 24 years
5	21	30	3	23	39	17	9	2	4	4	32	3	29	F	
17	26	33	3	65	97	44	19	7	7	7	43	5	44	M	25 - 34 years
10	32	38	5	84	79	33	27	9	17	7	48	9	45	F	
13	41	27	10	57	45	31	20	7	12	9	43	9	37	M	35 - 44 years
3	28	32	6	27	46	25	30	2	10	6	41	9	34	F	
17	29	20	6	39	47	25	26	6	13	8	52	11	36	M	45 - 54 years
13	23	15	3	45	35	9	18	3	13	4	58	6	25	F	
21	33	38	10	53	47	29	20	8	14	6	52	18	45	M	55 - 64 years
18	22	21	8	37	30	18	12	3	10	10	45	10	33	F	
25	30	57	8	49	34	26	10	19	15	15	49	14	39	M	65 - 74 years
6	20	24	6	25	15	15	3	6	9	8	29	8	21	F	
23	31	30	7	25	17	22	22	11	8	16	43	6	38	M	75 and over
18	16	16	6	22	19	20	18	11	8	5	37	9	26	F	
2	6	3	-	10	8	8	1	1	1	-	12	2	16	M	Unknown
1	1	3	1	4	6	4	3	-	-	1	5	2	6	F	
Tuberculosis, respiratory†															
105	**187**	**203**	**42**	**262**	**304**	**180**	**103**	**57**	**64**	**60**	**289**	**65**	**265**	M	All ages
65	**134**	**163**	**31**	**203**	**226**	**116**	**84**	**27**	**53**	**32**	**222**	**48**	**189**	F	
-	-	-	-	-	-	3	-	-	-	-	1	-	1	M	Under 1 year
-	-	-	-	-	-	-	-	-	1	-	1	-	-	F	
-	2	-	-	1	2	1	1	-	-	-	2	-	1	M	1 year
-	-	-	1	1	1	-	-	-	-	1	1	-	3	F	
1	2	-	-	2	2	4	2	1	1	-	4	1	9	M	2 - 4 years
-	5	6	-	3	3	1	1	-	1	-	5	3	9	F	
1	7	5	-	-	6	2	1	-	1	1	7	1	9	M	5 - 9 years
2	2	1	1	4	5	5	2	-	3	-	3	1	11	F	
3	5	1	-	3	3	4	-	1	1	-	9	-	11	M	10 - 14 years
2	3	4	1	7	7	1	-	1	1	-	7	-	5	F	
-	7	7	3	5	13	6	3	1	1	2	14	1	7	M	15 - 19 years
2	6	6	1	8	8	5	-	-	-	-	17	3	16	F	
-	11	14	2	26	29	3	3	3	7	1	24	4	14	M	20 - 24 years
3	17	24	3	14	28	11	6	2	2	2	22	2	16	F	
13	16	29	3	44	84	35	13	6	3	6	29	4	35	M	25 - 34 years
8	24	31	4	60	57	24	15	6	10	6	31	7	27	F	
11	28	23	6	34	35	26	17	4	9	9	30	8	27	M	35 - 44 years
2	20	24	4	16	32	18	17	2	4	6	22	6	21	F	
14	24	12	6	31	38	23	21	6	11	8	37	11	29	M	45 - 54 years
10	14	13	3	31	27	5	12	2	9	2	33	4	14	F	
16	27	30	8	45	39	24	13	7	11	5	38	16	38	M	55 - 64 years
15	13	19	5	20	25	15	10	2	6	5	31	7	24	F	
22	27	49	7	42	33	24	9	17	12	15	44	14	34	M	65 - 74 years
5	16	20	4	19	11	14	3	4	8	5	22	5	18	F	
22	25	30	7	19	13	21	19	10	6	13	42	3	36	M	75 and over
15	13	12	4	16	16	16	15	8	8	4	24	8	20	F	
2	6	3	-	10	7	4	1	1	1	-	8	2	14	M	Unknown
1	1	3	-	4	6	1	3	-	-	1	3	2	5	F	

Table 4 Series MB2 no.17

Table 4 - *continued*

Age-group	Sex	England and Wales (excluding port health authorities)	Wales	Standard regions								
				North	Yorkshire and Humberside	East Midlands	East Anglia	South East	South West	West Midlands	North West
Tuberculosis, meningitis*											
All ages	M	37	1	-	3	4	2	19	1	5	2
	F	44	3	2	2	4	1	18	2	5	7
Under 1 year	M	-	-	-	-	-	-	-	-	-	-
	F	-	-	-	-	-	-	-	-	-	-
1 year	M	1	-	-	-	-	-	-	-	1	-
	F	-	-	-	-	-	-	-	-	-	-
2 - 4 years	M	2	-	-	-	-	-	2	-	-	-
	F	2	-	-	-	-	1	-	1	-	-
5 - 9 years	M	1	1	-	-	-	-	-	-	-	-
	F	-	-	-	-	-	-	-	-	-	-
10 - 14 years	M	-	-	-	-	-	-	-	-	-	-
	F	1	-	-	-	-	-	-	-	-	1
15 - 19 years	M	2	-	-	1	1	-	-	-	-	-
	F	2	-	-	-	1	-	1	-	-	-
20 - 24 years	M	3	-	-	-	-	-	2	-	1	-
	F	5	-	1	1	-	-	1	-	-	2
25 - 34 years	M	4	-	-	1	1	-	1	-	-	1
	F	5	-	-	-	1	-	3	-	1	-
35 - 44 years	M	4	-	-	-	1	1	2	-	-	-
	F	5	-	-	1	-	-	3	-	-	1
45 - 54 years	M	6	-	-	-	1	-	3	-	1	1
	F	6	2	-	-	-	-	2	-	1	1
55 - 64 years	M	3	-	-	-	-	-	1	1	1	-
	F	6	1	-	-	-	-	3	-	1	1
65 - 74 years	M	7	-	-	1	-	1	4	-	1	-
	F	4	-	1	-	1	-	2	-	-	-
75 and over	M	3	-	-	-	-	-	3	-	-	-
	F	8	-	-	-	1	-	3	1	2	1
Unknown	M	1	-	-	-	-	-	1	-	-	-
	F	-	-	-	-	-	-	-	-	-	-
Tuberculosis, other forms†											
All ages	M	553	13	18	68	32	7	241	9	95	70
	F	675	14	15	75	35	15	270	22	129	100
Under 1 year	M	1	-	-	-	-	-	-	-	-	1
	F	4	-	-	-	-	1	1	-	1	1
1 year	M	3	-	-	-	-	1	2	-	-	-
	F	7	1	-	1	1	1	1	-	2	-
2 - 4 years	M	23	1	-	5	2	-	5	-	4	6
	F	16	1	1	6	-	-	3	-	2	3
5 - 9 years	M	21	-	-	1	-	1	10	1	3	5
	F	18	1	1	2	-	-	7	1	3	3
10 - 14 years	M	17	1	-	1	1	-	8	-	4	2
	F	26	-	-	4	2	-	7	-	7	6
15 - 19 years	M	21	-	-	2	2	-	7	1	7	2
	F	28	-	-	4	4	1	9	-	7	3
20 - 24 years	M	52	-	-	9	1	-	26	-	10	6
	F	65	-	1	6	5	-	29	2	10	12
25 - 34 years	M	98	3	4	11	4	-	50	2	15	9
	F	137	1	2	12	8	1	72	3	17	21
35 - 44 years	M	94	2	2	13	3	3	47	-	13	11
	F	106	1	1	10	7	2	50	-	20	15
45 - 54 years	M	64	2	3	8	4	-	24	-	17	6
	F	92	1	3	10	1	-	36	2	27	12
55 - 64 years	M	77	1	5	8	8	2	29	1	13	10
	F	77	-	3	12	1	4	27	6	13	11
65 - 74 years	M	39	3	3	4	7	-	13	-	4	5
	F	41	4	-	4	3	2	11	4	7	6
75 and over	M	32	-	1	6	-	-	15	4	1	5
	F	50	4	3	4	3	2	13	4	11	6
Unknown	M	11	-	-	-	-	-	5	-	4	2
	F	8	-	-	-	-	1	4	-	2	1

* Specificity codes 23.3, .5, .7.
† Specificity codes 23.4, .6, .8.

Northern	York-shire	Trent	East Anglian	North West Thames	North East Thames	South East Thames	South West Thames	Wessex	Oxford	South Western	West Midlands	Mersey	North Western	Sex	Age-group
Regional health authorities														Sex	Age-group
Tuberculosis, meningitis*															
-	3	3	2	2	4	4	2	-	8	1	5	-	2	M	All ages
2	2	4	1	1	6	2	2	1	7	1	5	-	7	F	
-	-	-	-	-	-	-	-	-	-	-	-	-	-	M	Under 1 year
-	-	-	-	-	-	-	-	-	-	-	-	-	-	F	
-	-	-	-	-	-	-	-	-	-	-	1	-	-	M	1 year
-	-	-	-	-	-	-	-	-	-	-	-	-	-	F	
-	-	-	-	-	1	-	-	-	1	-	-	-	-	M	2 - 4 years
-	-	-	1	-	-	-	-	-	-	1	-	-	-	F	
-	-	-	-	-	-	-	-	-	-	-	-	-	-	M	5 - 9 years
-	-	-	-	-	-	-	-	-	-	-	-	-	-	F	
-	-	-	-	-	-	-	-	-	-	-	-	-	-	M	10 - 14 years
-	-	-	-	-	-	-	-	-	-	-	-	-	1	F	
-	1	1	-	-	-	-	-	-	-	-	-	-	-	M	15 - 19 years
-	-	1	-	-	-	-	-	-	1	-	-	-	-	F	
-	-	-	-	2	-	-	-	-	-	-	1	-	-	M	20 - 24 years
1	1	-	-	-	-	-	1	-	-	-	-	-	2	F	
-	1	-	-	-	-	-	-	-	2	-	-	-	1	M	25 - 34 years
-	-	1	-	-	2	-	-	-	1	-	1	-	-	F	
-	-	1	1	-	1	1	-	-	-	-	-	-	-	M	35 - 44 years
-	1	-	-	1	1	-	-	-	1	-	-	-	1	F	
-	-	1	-	-	1	1	1	-	-	-	1	-	1	M	45 - 54 years
-	-	-	-	-	1	-	-	-	1	-	1	-	1	F	
-	-	-	-	-	-	1	-	-	-	1	1	-	-	M	55 - 64 years
-	-	-	-	-	1	-	-	-	2	-	1	-	1	F	
-	1	-	1	-	-	-	1	-	3	-	1	-	-	M	65 - 74 years
1	-	1	-	-	1	-	-	-	1	-	-	-	-	F	
-	-	-	-	-	1	-	-	-	2	-	-	-	-	M	75 and over
-	-	1	-	-	-	2	1	1	-	-	2	-	1	F	
-	-	-	-	1	-	-	-	-	-	-	-	-	-	M	Unknown
-	-	-	-	-	-	-	-	-	-	-	-	-	-	F	
Tuberculosis, other forms†															
18	57	41	7	90	63	38	29	12	15	5	95	11	59	M	All ages
15	61	42	15	94	72	43	41	15	19	15	129	16	84	F	
-	-	-	-	-	-	-	-	-	-	-	-	-	1	M	Under 1 year
-	-	-	1	-	-	1	-	-	-	-	1	-	1	F	
-	-	-	1	-	-	2	-	-	-	-	-	-	-	M	1 year
-	1	1	1	-	1	-	-	-	-	-	2	-	-	F	
-	4	3	-	1	2	1	-	-	1	-	4	1	5	M	2 - 4 years
1	4	2	-	-	-	1	-	2	-	-	2	-	3	F	
-	1	-	1	3	4	3	-	-	-	1	3	1	4	M	5 - 9 years
1	1	1	-	1	3	1	-	2	-	1	3	-	3	F	
-	-	2	-	1	3	1	1	2	-	-	4	-	2	M	10 - 14 years
-	3	3	-	3	1	3	-	-	-	-	7	-	6	F	
-	2	2	-	1	2	3	1	1	-	-	7	-	2	M	15 - 19 years
-	4	3	1	1	2	2	3	1	1	-	7	1	2	F	
-	8	2	-	8	9	3	2	1	3	-	10	1	5	M	20 - 24 years
1	4	6	-	9	11	6	2	-	2	2	10	1	11	F	
4	9	5	-	21	13	9	6	1	2	1	15	1	8	M	25 - 34 years
2	10	8	1	25	21	9	12	3	6	1	17	2	19	F	
2	13	3	3	25	9	4	3	3	3	-	13	1	10	M	35 - 44 years
1	7	8	2	11	16	7	13	-	5	-	20	3	12	F	
3	5	7	-	8	8	1	5	-	2	-	17	-	6	M	45 - 54 years
3	9	2	-	15	7	4	6	1	3	2	27	2	10	F	
5	6	9	2	8	8	4	7	1	3	-	13	3	7	M	55 - 64 years
3	10	2	4	17	4	3	2	1	2	5	13	3	8	F	
3	3	8	-	7	1	2	-	2	1	-	4	-	5	M	65 - 74 years
-	4	3	2	6	3	1	-	2	-	3	7	3	3	F	
1	6	-	-	7	4	1	3	1	-	3	13	3	2	M	75 and over
3	4	3	2	6	3	2	2.	3	-	1	11	1	5	F	
-	-	-	-	-	-	4	1	-	-	-	4	-	2	M	Unknown
-	-	-	1	-	-	3	1	-	-	-	2	-	1	F	

Table 4 Series MB2 no.17

Table 4 - *continued*

Age-group	Sex	England and Wales (excluding port health authorities)	Wales	Standard regions							
				North	Yorkshire and Humberside	East Midlands	East Anglia	South East	South West	West Midlands	North West
Whooping cough											
All ages	**M**	**7,075**	**551**	**687**	**916**	**459**	**242**	**1,917**	**595**	**666**	**1,042**
	F	**8,211**	**610**	**843**	**1,113**	**477**	**266**	**2,066**	**686**	**791**	**1,359**
Under 3 months	M	173	19	14	24	8	7	47	17	11	26
	F	207	16	25	26	16	6	45	18	9	46
3 - 5 months	M	289	33	25	33	15	6	72	15	34	56
	F	270	29	24	38	18	7	64	19	20	51
6 - 8 months	M	179	15	18	26	11	3	42	18	21	25
	F	185	22	10	25	6	6	50	11	19	36
9 - 11 months	M	134	10	10	18	5	7	44	6	15	19
	F	155	6	19	15	8	7	35	14	16	35
1 year	M	581	53	50	71	31	8	161	49	56	102
	F	606	47	69	80	26	17	136	52	66	113
2 years	M	726	64	62	87	42	27	197	62	72	113
	F	870	92	87	106	48	25	195	62	88	167
3 years	M	775	61	90	111	55	20	182	65	69	122
	F	925	78	89	129	51	27	213	74	82	182
4 years	M	804	78	79	95	46	32	182	71	86	135
	F	880	80	88	109	54	21	204	83	79	162
5 years	M	814	79	76	111	40	21	209	71	89	118
	F	971	65	103	141	52	38	246	79	97	150
6 years	M	747	45	73	102	60	32	197	66	59	113
	F	870	55	97	112	46	35	236	83	87	119
7 years	M	456	29	65	60	31	13	128	34	39	57
	F	574	37	58	82	27	17	149	51	64	89
8 years	M	306	12	24	38	19	17	102	35	26	33
	F	356	19	40	52	26	13	92	28	33	53
9 years	M	235	10	32	28	17	11	70	25	21	21
	F	336	13	39	40	39	14	88	33	32	38
10 - 14 years	M	481	20	45	67	56	25	143	30	40	55
	F	521	25	49	91	43	17	156	40	42	58
15 - 19 years	M	70	4	6	4	4	4	25	6	4	13
	F	77	4	12	12	-	1	22	5	13	8
20 - 24 years	M	32	1	1	4	2	-	17	1	2	4
	F	39	3	1	5	-	3	20	4	2	1
25 - 34 years	M	66	3	5	10	1	2	27	6	4	8
	F	122	5	8	22	8	4	39	11	12	13
35 - 44 years	M	62	4	8	5	5	1	26	4	5	4
	F	88	3	7	4	2	3	38	6	13	12
45 - 54 years	M	24	1	1	3	4	1	7	2	2	3
	F	38	2	6	6	3	1	7	3	4	6
55 - 64 years	M	13	-	-	1	2	-	8	-	1	1
	F	17	2	3	3	-	-	4	2	1	2
65 - 74 years	M	4	2	-	-	-	-	1	-	-	1
	F	14	1	1	1	-	-	6	3	1	1
75 and over	M	3	1	-	-	-	-	2	-	-	-
	F	3	-	-	-	-	-	-	-	1	2
Unknown	M	101	7	3	18	5	5	28	12	10	13
	F	87	6	8	14	4	4	21	5	10	15

North-ern	York-shire	Trent	East Anglian	North West Thames	North East Thames	South East Thames	South West Thames	Wessex	Oxford	South West-ern	West Mid-lands	Mersey	North West-ern	Sex	Age-group
Regional health authorities														Sex	Age-group

Whooping cough

North-ern	York-shire	Trent	East Anglian	North West Thames	North East Thames	South East Thames	South West Thames	Wessex	Oxford	South West-ern	West Mid-lands	Mersey	North West-ern	Sex	Age-group
687	**706**	**604**	**242**	**344**	**446**	**446**	**296**	**327**	**272**	**446**	**666**	**418**	**624**	M	All ages
843	**876**	**645**	**266**	**381**	**474**	**523**	**297**	**349**	**281**	**516**	**791**	**530**	**829**	F	
14	18	13	7	7	12	10	9	7	6	14	11	8	18	M	Under 3 months
25	20	18	6	11	5	11	7	15	9	9	9	21	25	F	
25	24	22	6	12	22	19	8	9	9	10	34	33	23	M	3 - 5 months
24	32	23	7	9	15	16	8	15	9	12	20	17	34	F	
18	24	10	3	6	12	9	4	12	7	13	21	8	17	M	6 - 8 months
10	18	13	6	9	12	8	11	12	3	6	19	14	22	F	
10	7	15	7	6	11	8	9	4	8	5	15	9	10	M	9 - 11 months
19	14	8	7	6	8	11	7	2	3	13	16	11	24	F	
50	56	46	8	27	39	41	17	32	20	34	56	41	61	M	1 year
69	61	40	17	26	35	29	14	32	20	37	66	51	62	F	
62	71	52	27	37	42	52	28	37	25	44	72	45	68	M	2 years
87	88	58	25	41	45	53	21	34	23	48	88	62	105	F	
90	96	64	20	39	34	44	27	28	27	54	69	50	72	M	3 years
89	104	67	27	56	44	58	29	25	22	62	82	68	114	F	
79	76	56	32	30	45	36	37	36	22	56	86	51	84	M	4 years
88	84	69	21	35	51	52	23	39	35	62	79	63	99	F	
76	81	63	21	34	54	50	24	27	35	63	89	40	78	M	5 years
103	117	69	38	42	51	60	28	52	42	57	97	56	94	F	
73	70	77	32	30	48	55	29	41	29	46	59	47	66	M	6 years
97	93	62	35	36	62	53	43	31	32	65	87	47	72	F	
65	47	40	13	28	32	26	18	18	21	23	39	21	36	M	7 years
58	62	43	17	26	36	30	25	27	23	37	64	33	56	F	
24	30	25	17	21	14	21	21	26	15	21	26	15	18	M	8 years
40	39	36	13	13	22	22	18	16	12	20	33	20	33	F	
32	21	20	11	17	13	14	13	10	13	19	21	7	14	M	9 years
39	26	48	14	17	23	24	12	13	10	27	32	14	24	F	
45	47	71	25	24	27	31	27	21	26	22	40	17	38	M	10 - 14 years
49	65	62	17	27	34	42	26	17	24	33	42	27	31	F	
6	3	5	4	5	7	5	3	5	2	4	4	6	7	M	15 - 19 years
12	11	1	1	2	3	8	4	1	4	5	13	3	5	F	
1	3	3	-	5	4	5	1	2	1	-	2	2	2	M	20 - 24 years
1	4	1	3	4	2	9	2	1	2	4	2	1	-	F	
5	8	3	2	6	7	3	8	2	2	5	4	5	3	M	25 - 34 years
8	17	12	4	8	9	12	6	6	3	7	12	8	5	F	
8	4	6	1	5	11	2	5	2	1	4	5	2	2	M	35 - 44 years
7	2	3	3	7	9	11	7	4	3	4	13	3	9	F	
1	3	4	1	3	-	2	2	-	-	2	2	2	1	M	45 - 54 years
6	5	4	1	1	2	1	1	2	2	1	4	5	1	F	
-	1	2	-	-	1	2	2	1	2	-	1	-	1	M	55 - 64 years
3	1	2	-	1	-	2	1	-	-	2	1	1	1	F	
-	-	-	-	-	-	1	-	-	-	-	-	1	-	M	65 - 74 years
1	1	-	-	1	-	1	3	2	-	2	1	1	-	F	
-	-	-	-	-	-	2	-	-	-	-	-	-	-	M	75 and over
-	-	-	-	-	-	-	-	-	-	-	1	-	2	F	
3	16	7	5	2	11	8	4	7	1	7	10	8	5	M	Unknown
8	12	6	4	3	6	10	1	3	-	3	10	4	11	F	

Table 4 Series MB2 no.17

Table 4 - *continued*

Age-group	Sex	England and Wales (excluding port health authorities)	Wales	Standard regions							
				North	Yorkshire and Humberside	East Midlands	East Anglia	South East	South West	West Midlands	North West
Scarlet fever											
All ages	M	**3,501**	**95**	**227**	**667**	**294**	**85**	**1,076**	**304**	**383**	**370**
	F	**3,686**	**104**	**211**	**693**	**309**	**101**	**1,122**	**291**	**441**	**414**
Under 1 year	M	50	3	5	9	2	1	10	5	9	6
	F	54	3	5	5	4	1	17	2	10	7
1 year	M	140	-	13	26	5	3	44	12	19	18
	F	129	3	8	21	8	3	50	9	13	14
2 years	M	248	5	14	31	24	5	83	29	32	25
	F	211	5	13	40	14	8	56	15	29	31
3 years	M	401	10	25	72	28	9	133	29	48	47
	F	394	10	26	66	29	12	133	31	45	42
4 years	M	548	14	28	99	39	15	182	57	60	54
	F	490	14	30	94	36	11	164	35	52	54
5 years	M	525	15	42	93	43	16	173	42	53	48
	F	537	10	27	91	56	12	162	52	61	66
6 years	M	324	11	20	64	34	9	101	20	26	39
	F	377	8	27	88	34	9	104	29	44	34
7 years	M	180	4	9	34	19	2	51	21	21	19
	F	265	10	17	37	23	6	79	23	39	31
8 years	M	143	5	11	28	12	3	39	16	20	9
	F	188	4	8	47	12	4	51	17	24	21
9 years	M	112	5	7	34	9	4	30	6	9	8
	F	161	7	8	23	14	6	52	10	23	18
10 - 14 years	M	279	10	16	72	24	7	69	23	31	27
	F	308	15	14	76	33	11	80	18	27	34
15 - 24 years	M	333	7	27	62	34	4	91	27	41	40
	F	266	7	12	50	25	7	68	32	36	29
25 - 44 years	M	153	6	7	30	16	4	47	11	9	23
	F	223	7	13	39	18	9	80	13	25	19
45 and over	M	16	-	1	3	1	-	7	3	-	1
	F	33	1	2	2	2	1	9	2	6	8
Unknown	M	49	-	2	10	4	3	16	3	5	6
	F	50	-	1	14	1	1	17	3	7	6
Meningitis, all forms											
All ages	M	**1,347**	**113**	**65**	**179**	**84**	**40**	**372**	**128**	**133**	**233**
	F	**1,225**	**90**	**81**	**165**	**79**	**36**	**355**	**104**	**129**	**186**
Under 1 year	M	328	25	22	43	20	8	86	31	36	57
	F	277	24	23	35	14	5	88	14	30	44
1 year	M	196	16	10	19	5	9	66	13	21	37
	F	151	8	13	19	17	5	36	10	20	23
2 years	M	95	12	4	9	6	-	25	9	8	22
	F	84	5	3	9	6	3	31	5	6	16
3 years	M	73	4	5	7	9	2	17	9	12	8
	F	54	7	5	7	2	1	15	1	5	11
4 years	M	41	7	2	4	1	2	9	5	5	6
	F	32	3	3	2	1	-	6	4	7	6
5 - 9 years	M	118	10	4	16	7	6	23	13	10	29
	F	84	5	4	13	5	2	21	6	5	23
10 - 14 years	M	74	5	3	14	3	5	11	8	7	18
	F	66	6	6	8	2	3	13	6	10	12
15 - 24 years	M	187	14	4	32	16	3	55	22	14	27
	F	162	11	9	27	5	6	52	21	15	16
25 and over	M	207	19	11	30	14	3	75	16	14	25
	F	286	20	15	40	23	5	88	37	27	31
Unknown	M	28	1	-	5	3	2	5	2	6	4
	F	29	1	-	5	4	6	5	-	4	4

Northern	York-shire	Trent	East Anglian	North West Thames	North East Thames	South East Thames	South West Thames	Wessex	Oxford	South West-ern	West Mid-lands	Mersey	North West-ern	Sex	Age-group
Scarlet fever															
227	**515**	**421**	**85**	**196**	**254**	**264**	**167**	**176**	**140**	**208**	**383**	**181**	**189**	M	All ages
211	**520**	**445**	**101**	**197**	**288**	**261**	**183**	**175**	**158**	**188**	**441**	**197**	**217**	F	
5	8	3	1	1	4	1	3	2	1	3	9	2	4	M	Under 1 year
5	5	1	1	1	7	4	2	-	6	2	10	1	6	F	
13	21	10	3	9	12	13	5	6	4	7	19	6	12	M	1 year
8	19	9	3	9	9	20	7	6	4	5	13	6	8	F	
14	27	24	5	17	19	19	17	15	11	18	32	14	11	M	2 years
13	25	27	8	6	19	8	12	7	12	9	29	11	20	F	
25	63	36	9	26	33	33	23	21	12	15	48	24	23	M	3 years
26	50	41	12	26	30	38	23	16	14	21	45	19	23	F	
28	70	64	15	26	40	44	35	31	26	41	60	27	27	M	4 years
30	66	61	11	35	40	41	19	25	22	20	52	30	24	F	
42	68	62	16	28	44	40	20	26	34	29	53	20	28	M	5 years
27	68	71	12	25	35	39	34	26	28	35	61	27	39	F	
20	48	48	9	20	19	32	15	17	10	10	26	22	17	M	6 years
27	76	43	9	19	39	17	13	11	15	22	44	17	17	F	
9	24	29	2	11	14	11	8	10	3	15	21	14	5	M	7 years
17	26	32	6	14	15	15	16	12	14	18	39	18	13	F	
11	23	17	3	8	10	7	6	8	5	11	20	7	2	M	8 years
8	31	28	4	7	10	10	13	7	9	12	24	14	7	F	
7	27	15	4	7	6	3	3	5	7	6	9	5	3	M	9 years
8	15	22	6	9	16	10	8	10	3	6	23	12	6	F	
16	57	37	7	15	13	22	6	10	11	17	31	13	14	M	10 - 14 years
14	55	52	11	15	25	16	13	12	7	12	27	19	15	F	
27	47	45	4	20	19	16	18	17	9	23	41	17	23	M	15 - 24 years
12	39	33	7	11	13	16	11	25	9	18	36	13	16	F	
7	23	22	4	5	13	15	7	3	7	9	9	10	13	M	25 - 44 years
13	32	19	9	13	24	20	11	13	12	6	25	6	13	F	
1	1	3	-	2	1	3	1	1	-	2	-	-	1	M	45 and over
2	2	2	1	4	2	-	1	1	2	1	6	4	4	F	
2	8	6	3	1	7	5	-	4	-	2	5	-	6	M	Unknown
1	11	4	1	3	4	7	-	4	1	1	7	-	6	F	
Meningitis, all forms															
65	**135**	**113**	**40**	**69**	**89**	**88**	**54**	**57**	**51**	**107**	**133**	**88**	**145**	M	All ages
81	**119**	**109**	**36**	**70**	**79**	**80**	**51**	**50**	**64**	**81**	**129**	**74**	**112**	F	
22	30	28	8	12	19	27	11	15	15	23	36	16	41	M	Under 1 year
23	24	20	5	15	18	20	12	8	24	10	30	17	27	F	
10	14	10	9	11	13	15	13	9	9	9	21	14	23	M	1 year
13	11	23	5	7	8	13	-	7	7	6	20	6	17	F	
4	8	6	-	6	4	7	3	7	2	6	8	11	11	M	2 years
3	8	7	3	4	9	9	3	3	3	5	6	5	11	F	
5	6	10	2	-	4	7	3	3	1	8	12	5	3	M	3 years
5	6	3	1	4	4	4	1	1	1	1	5	5	6	F	
2	4	1	2	1	4	3	1	-	-	5	5	3	3	M	4 years
3	2	1	-	-	1	3	-	3	1	2	7	4	2	F	
4	14	9	6	2	9	3	5	3	3	11	10	11	18	M	5 - 9 years
4	11	7	2	1	10	6	3	2	1	4	5	9	14	F	
3	12	4	5	3	4	3	1	-	1	8	7	6	12	M	10 - 14 years
6	8	1	3	5	3	2	-	1	4	5	10	6	6	F	
4	23	23	3	17	14	8	4	10	6	20	14	8	19	M	15 - 24 years
9	22	9	6	14	9	7	9	7	9	19	15	7	9	F	
11	20	18	3	16	18	14	13	8	13	15	14	13	12	M	25 and over
15	23	35	5	19	16	15	21	18	12	29	27	13	18	F	
-	4	4	2	1	-	1	-	2	1	2	6	1	3	M	Unknown
-	4	3	6	1	1	1	2	-	2	-	4	2	2	F	

Table 4 Series MB2 no.17

Table 4 - *continued*

Age-group	Sex	England and Wales (excluding port health authorities)	Wales	Standard regions							
				North	Yorkshire and Humberside	East Midlands	East Anglia	South East	South West	West Midlands	North West
Meningitis, meningococcal											
All ages	M	**605**	**41**	**36**	**81**	**42**	**15**	**155**	**60**	**55**	**120**
	F	**533**	**30**	**40**	**55**	**35**	**19**	**162**	**40**	**61**	**91**
Under 1 year	M	134	7	15	21	7	3	27	9	13	32
	F	112	9	7	9	7	3	36	8	9	24
1 year	M	78	7	5	7	3	-	22	6	10	18
	F	62	2	6	6	6	1	15	3	11	12
2 years	M	46	7	3	7	2	-	12	2	4	9
	F	38	2	2	2	3	2	17	-	2	8
3 years	M	27	1	1	2	2	1	6	5	4	5
	F	29	3	3	3	2	-	8	-	3	7
4 years	M	23	3	1	2	1	1	4	3	3	5
	F	10	1	2	-	-	-	4	1	-	2
5 - 9 years	M	59	4	3	6	5	2	14	8	1	16
	F	44	3	2	4	1	1	12	5	4	12
10 - 14 years	M	33	4	2	6	1	3	3	3	2	9
	F	38	1	3	5	2	2	8	4	6	7
15 - 24 years	M	124	4	2	23	14	3	41	16	8	13
	F	98	4	8	15	4	4	31	13	8	11
25 and over	M	68	4	4	4	6	1	25	6	6	12
	F	91	4	7	11	8	4	28	6	15	8
Unknown	M	13	-	-	3	1	1	1	2	4	1
	F	11	1	-	-	2	2	3	-	3	-
Meningitis, pneumococcal											
All ages	M	**87**	**7**	**4**	**9**	**1**	**4**	**36**	**6**	**9**	**11**
	F	**69**	**6**	**6**	**7**	**10**	**1**	**20**	**4**	**8**	**7**
Under 1 year	M	23	-	1	3	1	1	11	2	3	1
	F	14	1	2	2	-	-	5	-	2	2
1 year	M	10	1	-	2	-	1	4	1	-	1
	F	5	-	-	1	1	-	1	1	1	-
2 years	M	3	-	-	-	-	-	1	1	-	1
	F	3	-	-	1	-	-	1	-	1	-
3 years	M	4	-	-	1	-	1	1	-	-	1
	F	2	1	-	-	-	-	1	-	-	-
4 years	M	1	1	-	-	-	-	-	-	-	-
	F	2	-	1	-	-	-	1	-	-	-
5 - 9 years	M	4	1	-	-	-	1	-	1	-	1
	F	3	-	-	-	2	-	1	-	-	-
10 - 14 years	M	1	-	-	-	-	-	-	-	1	-
	F	1	-	-	1	-	-	-	-	-	-
15 - 24 years	M	5	1	-	-	-	-	2	-	-	2
	F	1	-	-	1	-	-	-	-	-	-
25 and over	M	35	2	3	3	-	-	17	1	5	4
	F	35	4	3	1	7	-	10	3	4	3
Unknown	M	1	1	-	-	-	-	-	-	-	-
	F	3	-	-	-	-	1	-	-	-	2
Meningitis, influenzal (Haemophilus influenzae)											
All ages	M	**220**	**17**	**9**	**16**	**18**	**10**	**70**	**21**	**27**	**32**
	F	**211**	**16**	**14**	**28**	**14**	**5**	**73**	**13**	**22**	**26**
Under 1 year	M	90	7	3	9	6	2	24	13	13	13
	F	67	3	4	7	4	1	30	2	10	6
1 year	M	58	5	3	5	1	4	23	3	5	9
	F	59	6	5	10	6	3	13	5	4	7
2 years	M	24	2	1	-	3	-	8	2	3	5
	F	32	2	1	4	3	-	11	2	2	7
3 years	M	24	3	1	-	5	-	8	3	3	1
	F	17	3	2	3	-	1	5	1	1	1
4 years	M	3	-	-	1	-	1	1	-	-	-
	F	7	1	-	-	-	-	-	3	2	1
5 - 9 years	M	7	-	-	1	-	2	1	-	2	1
	F	10	1	1	1	1	-	3	-	1	2
10 - 14 years	M	3	-	-	-	1	-	1	-	-	1
	F	2	-	1	-	-	-	1	-	-	-
15 - 24 years	M	2	-	-	-	-	-	1	-	-	1
	F	3	-	-	-	-	-	2	-	-	1
25 and over	M	5	-	1	-	2	-	2	-	-	-
	F	13	-	-	2	-	-	8	-	2	1
Unknown	M	4	-	-	-	-	1	1	-	1	1
	F	1	-	-	1	-	-	-	-	-	-

Northern	Yorkshire	Trent	East Anglian	North West Thames	North East Thames	South East Thames	South West Thames	Wessex	Oxford	South Western	West Midlands	Mersey	North Western	Sex	Age-group

Meningitis, meningococcal

Northern	Yorkshire	Trent	East Anglian	North West Thames	North East Thames	South East Thames	South West Thames	Wessex	Oxford	South Western	West Midlands	Mersey	North Western	Sex	Age-group
36	58	62	15	33	32	36	24	28	14	51	55	48	72	M	All ages
40	42	42	19	34	34	35	22	21	28	34	61	30	61	F	
15	15	13	3	1	8	11	3	4	2	7	13	11	21	M	Under 1 year
7	5	9	3	5	8	9	4	4	9	7	9	10	14	F	
5	5	5	-	6	3	6	4	3	2	4	10	5	13	M	1 year
6	4	7	1	3	3	4	-	2	3	2	11	2	10	F	
3	6	3	-	2	1	4	3	3	-	1	4	4	5	M	2 years
2	2	3	2	1	5	5	2	3	1	-	2	2	6	F	
1	1	3	1	-	-	1	3	2	-	5	4	3	2	M	3 years
3	3	2	-	1	2	3	-	1	1	-	3	4	3	F	
1	2	1	1	-	3	1	-	-	-	3	3	3	2	M	4 years
2	-	-	-	-	1	2	-	-	1	1	-	1	1	F	
3	4	7	2	1	3	2	5	3	2	6	1	6	10	M	5 - 9 years
2	4	1	1	1	3	5	2	2	1	3	4	4	8	F	
2	5	2	3	1	2	-	-	-	-	3	2	3	6	M	10 - 14 years
3	5	1	2	3	2	2	-	-	2	4	6	2	5	F	
2	15	20	3	14	8	6	3	9	5	14	8	5	8	M	15 - 24 years
8	13	6	4	11	5	3	7	2	4	12	8	4	7	F	
4	3	6	1	8	4	4	3	4	3	6	6	7	5	M	25 and over
7	6	12	4	6	4	2	6	7	5	5	15	1	7	F	
-	2	2	1	-	-	1	-	-	-	2	4	1	-	M	Unknown
-	-	1	2	1	1	-	1	-	1	-	3	-	-	F	

Meningitis, pneumococcal

Northern	Yorkshire	Trent	East Anglian	North West Thames	North East Thames	South East Thames	South West Thames	Wessex	Oxford	South Western	West Midlands	Mersey	North Western	Sex	Age-group
4	5	5	4	6	8	12	6	3	3	4	9	5	6	M	All ages
6	4	12	1	5	5	4	1	2	4	4	8	2	5	F	
1	2	2	1	-	2	4	3	1	1	2	3	-	1	M	Under 1 year
2	1	1	-	-	1	-	1	-	3	-	2	-	2	F	
-	-	2	1	1	-	3	-	-	-	1	-	1	-	M	1 year
-	1	1	-	1	-	-	-	-	-	1	1	-	-	F	
-	-	-	-	1	1	-	-	1	-	-	-	-	1	M	2 years
-	1	-	-	1	-	-	-	-	-	-	1	-	-	F	
-	1	-	1	-	-	1	-	-	-	-	-	1	-	M	3 years
-	-	-	1	-	-	-	-	-	-	-	-	-	-	F	
-	-	-	-	-	-	-	-	-	-	-	-	-	-	M	4 years
1	-	-	-	-	-	-	-	1	-	-	-	-	-	F	
-	-	-	1	-	-	-	-	-	-	1	-	1	-	M	5 - 9 years
-	-	2	-	-	-	1	-	-	-	-	-	-	-	F	
-	-	-	-	-	-	-	-	-	-	-	1	-	-	M	10 - 14 years
-	1	-	-	-	-	-	-	-	-	-	-	-	-	F	
-	-	-	-	1	-	-	-	-	1	-	-	-	2	M	15 - 24 years
-	-	1	-	-	-	-	-	-	-	-	-	-	-	F	
3	2	1	-	5	4	4	3	1	1	-	5	2	2	M	25 and over
3	-	7	-	3	3	3	-	1	1	3	4	1	2	F	
-	-	-	-	-	-	-	-	-	-	-	-	1	1	M	Unknown
-	-	-	1	-	-	-	-	-	-	-	-	1	1	F	

Meningitis, influenzal (Haemophilus influenzae)

Northern	Yorkshire	Trent	East Anglian	North West Thames	North East Thames	South East Thames	South West Thames	Wessex	Oxford	South Western	West Midlands	Mersey	North Western	Sex	Age-group
9	13	17	10	8	20	16	8	14	16	13	27	11	21	M	All ages
14	16	25	5	15	15	16	10	10	14	7	22	11	15	F	
3	6	7	2	5	4	8	2	7	5	8	13	2	11	M	Under 1 year
4	5	5	1	8	5	4	5	2	8	1	10	1	5	F	
3	5	1	4	1	7	1	5	3	7	2	5	4	5	M	1 year
5	4	12	3	-	3	7	-	5	1	2	4	4	3	F	
1	-	2	-	1	2	3	-	2	2	1	3	2	3	M	2 years
1	3	4	-	3	1	4	1	-	2	2	2	3	4	F	
1	-	5	-	-	4	3	-	1	1	2	3	1	-	M	3 years
2	2	1	1	1	2	1	1	-	-	1	1	1	-	F	4 years
-	1	-	1	-	1	-	-	-	2	-	-	-	-	M	
-	-	-	-	-	1	-	-	2	-	1	2	1	-	F	
-	1	-	2	-	-	1	-	-	-	-	2	1	-	M	5 - 9 years
1	-	2	-	-	2	-	1	-	-	-	1	-	2	F	
-	-	1	-	1	-	-	-	-	-	-	-	1	-	M	10 - 14 years
1	-	-	-	1	-	-	-	-	-	-	-	-	1	F	
-	-	-	-	1	-	-	-	-	1	-	-	-	1	M	15 - 24 years
-	-	-	-	1	-	-	-	-	1	-	-	-	1	F	
1	-	1	-	-	1	-	1	-	1	-	-	-	-	M	25 and over
-	1	1	-	1	2	-	2	1	2	-	2	1	1	F	
-	-	-	1	-	-	-	1	-	-	-	1	-	1	M	Unknown
-	1	-	-	-	-	-	-	-	-	-	-	-	-	F	

Table 4 Series MB2 no.17

Table 4 - *continued*

Age-group	Sex	England and Wales (excluding port health authorities)	Wales	Standard regions							
				North	Yorkshire and Humberside	East Midlands	East Anglia	South East	South West	West Midlands	North West
Meningitis, viral											
All ages	M	**166**	**8**	**6**	**48**	**11**	**3**	**43**	**14**	**12**	**21**
	F	**187**	**12**	**7**	**50**	**10**	**2**	**38**	**24**	**16**	**28**
Under 1 year	M	15	-	1	5	-	-	6	1	-	2
	F	20	3	2	7	1	-	3	1	-	3
1 year	M	9	-	-	2	-	1	1	1	2	2
	F	4	-	1	-	-	-	1	-	1	1
2 years	M	7	-	-	1	1	-	1	1	-	3
	F	2	-	-	1	-	-	-	-	1	-
3 years	M	6	-	1	1	1	-	1	-	2	-
	F	3	-	-	1	-	-	-	-	1	1
4 years	M	7	-	1	1	-	-	3	1	1	-
	F	4	1	-	1	-	-	-	-	1	1
5 - 9 years	M	25	1	1	6	2	1	3	3	3	5
	F	14	1	1	5	-	-	1	1	-	5
10 - 14 years	M	20	1	1	7	1	-	5	1	1	3
	F	16	1	-	2	-	1	2	2	3	5
15 - 24 years	M	21	3	1	6	1	-	3	4	1	2
	F	31	3	1	8	1	-	8	4	4	2
25 and over	M	53	3	-	18	4	1	19	2	2	4
	F	89	3	2	24	7	1	23	16	4	9
Unknown	M	3	-	-	1	1	-	1	-	-	-
	F	4	-	-	1	1	-	-	-	1	1
Meningitis, other specified											
All ages	M	**112**	**22**	**4**	**12**	**5**	**3**	**32**	**8**	**9**	**17**
	F	**115**	**18**	**5**	**12**	**4**	**3**	**28**	**16**	**11**	**18**
Under 1 year	M	30	8	1	2	3	1	8	2	2	3
	F	39	8	3	7	1	-	6	2	7	5
1 year	M	15	2	-	1	1	1	5	-	2	3
	F	10	-	-	1	1	-	4	-	2	2
2 years	M	6	1	-	1	-	-	2	-	-	2
	F	4	1	-	-	-	1	-	1	-	1
3 years	M	3	-	1	1	1	-	-	-	-	-
	F	1	-	-	-	-	-	1	-	-	-
4 years	M	1	-	-	-	-	-	-	-	1	-
	F	-	-	-	-	-	-	-	-	-	-
5 - 9 years	M	9	-	-	1	-	-	4	-	2	2
	F	2	-	-	-	-	-	1	-	-	1
10 - 14 years	M	3	-	-	-	-	-	1	1	-	1
	F	3	2	-	-	-	-	1	-	-	-
15 - 24 years	M	12	2	-	2	-	-	3	-	1	4
	F	14	-	-	1	-	1	6	3	2	1
25 and over	M	28	9	2	3	-	1	7	5	-	1
	F	38	7	2	1	1	-	9	10	-	8
Unknown	M	5	-	-	1	-	-	2	-	1	1
	F	4	-	-	2	1	1	-	-	-	-
Meningitis, unspecified											
All ages	M	**157**	**18**	**6**	**13**	**7**	**5**	**36**	**19**	**21**	**32**
	F	**110**	**8**	**9**	**13**	**6**	**6**	**34**	**7**	**11**	**16**
Under 1 year	M	36	3	1	3	3	1	10	4	5	6
	F	25	-	5	3	1	1	8	1	2	4
1 year	M	26	1	2	2	-	2	11	2	2	4
	F	11	-	1	1	3	1	2	1	1	1
2 years	M	9	2	-	-	-	-	1	3	1	2
	F	5	-	-	1	-	-	2	2	-	-
3 years	M	9	-	1	2	-	-	1	1	3	1
	F	2	-	-	-	-	-	-	-	-	2
4 years	M	6	3	-	-	-	-	1	1	-	1
	F	9	-	-	1	1	-	1	-	4	2
5 - 9 years	M	14	4	-	2	-	-	1	1	2	4
	F	11	-	-	3	1	1	3	-	-	3
10 - 14 years	M	14	-	-	1	-	2	1	3	3	4
	F	6	2	2	-	-	-	1	-	1	-
15 - 24 years	M	23	4	1	1	1	-	5	2	4	5
	F	15	4	-	2	-	1	5	1	1	1
25 and over	M	18	1	1	2	2	-	5	2	1	4
	F	20	2	1	1	-	-	10	2	2	2
Unknown	M	2	-	-	-	1	-	-	-	-	1
	F	6	-	-	1	-	2	2	-	-	1

North-ern	York-shire	Trent	East Anglian	North West Thames	North East Thames	South East Thames	South West Thames	Wessex	Oxford	South West-ern	West Mid-lands	Mersey	North West-ern	Sex	Age-group
Regional health authorities														**Sex**	**Age-group**
Meningitis, viral															
6	36	20	3	7	7	9	10	3	10	14	12	13	8	M	All ages
7	41	14	2	11	5	9	6	5	10	21	16	15	13	F	
1	2	3	-	1	1	-	2	-	2	1	-	1	1	M	Under 1 year
2	7	1	-	-	1	1	1	-	-	1	-	1	2	F	
-	1	1	1	-	-	1	-	-	-	1	2	2	-	M	1 year
1	-	-	-	-	-	-	-	-	1	-	1	-	1	F	
-	1	1	-	1	-	-	-	-	-	1	-	2	1	M	2 years
-	1	-	-	-	-	-	-	-	-	-	1	-	-	F	
1	1	1	-	-	-	1	-	-	-	-	2	-	-	M	3 years
-	1	-	-	-	-	-	-	-	-	-	1	-	1	F	
1	1	-	-	-	-	2	1	-	-	1	1	-	-	M	4 years
-	1	-	-	-	-	-	-	-	-	-	1	1	-	F	
1	6	2	1	-	2	-	-	-	1	3	3	2	3	M	5 - 9 years
1	5	-	-	-	1	-	-	-	-	1	-	4	1	F	
1	7	-	-	1	2	1	1	-	1	1	1	2	1	M	10 - 14 years
-	2	-	1	1	-	-	-	1	1	1	3	4	1	F	
1	5	2	-	2	-	-	1	-	-	4	1	1	1	M	15 - 24 years
1	7	1	-	1	1	3	-	1	3	4	4	1	1	F	
-	11	9	1	2	2	4	5	2	6	2	2	3	1	M	25 and over
2	16	12	1	9	2	5	5	3	4	14	4	4	5	F	
-	1	1	-	-	-	-	-	1	-	-	-	-	-	M	Unknown
-	1	-	-	-	-	-	-	-	1	-	1	-	1	F	
Meningitis, other specified															
4	12	4	3	8	11	6	2	4	3	7	9	4	13	M	All ages
5	7	8	3	4	8	6	8	6	3	10	11	9	9	F	
1	2	2	1	3	3	1	-	1	2	1	2	1	2	M	Under 1 year
3	5	2	-	2	-	2	1	1	2	1	7	3	2	F	
-	1	1	1	1	2	1	1	-	-	-	2	-	3	M	1 year
-	1	1	-	-	2	2	-	-	-	-	2	-	2	F	
-	1	-	-	1	-	-	-	1	-	-	-	2	-	M	2 years
-	-	-	1	-	-	-	-	-	-	1	-	-	1	F	
1	1	1	-	-	-	-	-	-	-	-	-	-	-	M	3 years
-	-	-	1	-	-	-	-	-	-	-	-	-	-	F	
-	-	-	-	-	-	-	-	-	-	-	1	-	-	M	4 years
-	-	-	-	-	-	-	-	-	-	-	-	-	-	F	
-	1	-	-	-	4	-	-	-	-	-	2	-	2	M	5 - 9 years
-	-	-	-	-	1	-	-	-	-	-	-	1	-	F	
-	-	-	-	-	-	1	-	-	-	1	-	-	1	M	10 - 14 years
-	-	-	-	-	1	-	-	-	-	-	-	-	-	F	
-	2	-	-	-	-	1	-	1	-	-	1	1	3	M	15 - 24 years
-	-	1	1	1	2	-	2	1	1	2	2	1	-	F	
2	3	-	1	1	2	2	1	1	-	5	-	-	1	M	25 and over
2	-	2	-	-	2	2	5	4	-	6	-	4	4	F	
-	1	-	-	1	-	-	-	-	1	-	1	-	1	M	Unknown
-	1	2	1	-	-	-	-	-	1	-	-	-	-	F	
Meningitis, unspecified															
6	11	5	5	7	11	9	4	5	5	18	21	7	25	M	All ages
9	9	8	6	1	12	10	4	6	5	5	11	7	9	F	
1	3	1	1	2	1	3	1	2	3	4	5	1	5	M	Under 1 year
5	1	2	1	-	3	4	-	1	2	-	2	2	2	F	
2	2	-	2	2	1	3	3	3	-	1	2	-	2	M	1 year
1	1	2	1	1	-	-	-	-	2	1	1	-	1	F	
-	-	-	-	1	-	-	-	-	-	3	1	1	1	M	2 years
-	1	-	-	-	2	-	-	-	-	2	-	-	-	F	
1	2	-	-	-	-	1	-	-	-	1	3	-	1	M	3 years
-	-	-	-	-	-	-	-	-	-	-	-	-	2	F	
-	-	-	-	1	-	-	1	-	-	1	-	-	1	M	4 years
-	1	1	-	-	-	1	-	-	-	-	4	1	1	F	
-	2	-	-	1	-	-	-	-	-	1	2	1	3	M	5 - 9 years
-	2	2	1	-	3	-	-	-	-	-	-	-	3	F	
-	-	1	2	-	-	1	-	-	-	3	3	-	4	M	10 - 14 years
2	-	-	-	-	-	-	-	-	1	-	1	-	-	F	
1	1	1	-	-	4	1	-	-	-	2	4	1	4	M	15 - 24 years
-	2	-	1	-	1	1	-	3	-	1	1	1	-	F	
1	1	1	-	-	5	-	-	-	2	2	1	1	3	M	25 and over
1	-	1	-	-	3	3	3	2	-	1	2	2	-	F	
-	-	1	-	-	-	-	-	-	-	-	-	-	1	M	Unknown
-	1	-	2	-	-	1	1	-	-	-	-	1	-	F	

Table 4 Series MB2 no.17

Table 4 - *continued*

Age-group	Sex	England and Wales (excluding port health authorities)	Wales	Standard regions							
				North	Yorkshire and Humberside	East Midlands	East Anglia	South East	South West	West Midlands	North West
Meningococcal septicaemia (without meningitis)											
All ages	**M**	**147**	**11**	**8**	**20**	**8**	**4**	**44**	**7**	**14**	**31**
	F	**130**	**11**	**11**	**13**	**10**	**2**	**33**	**15**	**9**	**26**
Under 1 year	M	36	2	3	7	2	-	10	1	1	10
	F	28	2	2	4	3	1	5	1	3	7
1 year	M	21	2	1	4	2	-	3	1	3	5
	F	22	3	-	2	3	1	3	4	1	5
2 years	M	18	-	-	2	1	-	8	1	1	5
	F	9	1	-	1	2	-	3	-	-	2
3 years	M	6	-	-	-	-	-	4	-	-	2
	F	6	-	2	1	-	-	-	1	1	1
4 years	M	6	1	2	1	-	-	1	-	-	1
	F	7	1	1	2	1	-	1	-	-	1
5 - 9 years	M	18	1	1	3	-	-	4	2	2	5
	F	13	-	3	1	-	-	2	2	2	3
10 - 14 years	M	9	1	-	-	1	2	2	1	-	2
	F	8	-	-	-	-	-	4	1	-	3
15 - 24 years	M	19	3	-	2	1	1	8	1	2	1
	F	11	-	-	2	-	-	8	1	-	-
25 and over	M	11	1	1	1	1	-	2	-	5	-
	F	24	4	3	-	-	-	6	5	2	4
Unknown	M	3	-	-	-	-	1	2	-	-	-
	F	2	-	-	-	1	-	1	-	-	-

Regional health authorities														Sex	Age-group
North- ern	York- shire	Trent	East Anglian	North West Thames	North East Thames	South East Thames	South West Thames	Wessex	Oxford	South West- ern	West Mid- lands	Mersey	North West- ern		
Meningococcal septicaemia (without meningitis)															
8	**13**	**14**	**4**	**10**	**10**	**5**	**5**	**4**	**12**	**6**	**14**	**17**	**14**	M	**All ages**
11	**13**	**7**	**2**	**7**	**7**	**4**	**7**	**3**	**8**	**15**	**9**	**11**	**15**	F	
3	4	5	-	3	2	2	1	1	2	-	1	7	3	M	Under 1 year
2	4	2	1	1	2	-	1	1	1	1	3	3	4	F	
1	3	3	-	1	-	-	1	-	1	1	3	4	1	M	1 year
-	2	2	1	-	1	-	-	1	2	4	1	2	3	F	
-	2	1	-	2	1	1	1	2	1	1	1	2	3	M	2 years
-	1	2	-	1	-	-	2	-	-	-	-	1	1	F	
-	-	-	-	1	3	-	-	-	-	-	-	2	-	M	3 years
2	1	-	-	-	-	-	-	-	-	1	1	-	1	F	
2	-	1	-	-	-	-	-	-	1	-	-	-	1	M	4 years
1	2	1	-	1	-	-	-	-	-	-	-	-	1	F	
1	3	-	-	-	2	-	-	-	2	2	2	2	3	M	5 - 9 years
3	1	-	-	-	-	-	-	-	2	2	2	1	2	F	
-	-	1	2	1	-	-	-	-	1	1	-	-	2	M	10 - 14 years
-	-	-	1	1	-	-	1	-	2	1	-	1	2	F	
-	1	1	1	2	-	1	2	1	3	1	2	-	1	M	15 - 24 years
-	2	-	-	2	2	2	1	1	-	1	-	-	-	F	
1	-	2	-	-	1	-	-	-	1	-	5	3	-	M	25 and over
3	-	-	-	1	1	2	2	-	-	5	2	3	1	F	
-	-	-	1	-	1	1	-	-	-	-	-	-	-	M	Unknown
-	-	-	-	-	1	-	-	-	1	-	-	-	-	F	

Table 4 Series MB2 no.17

Table 4 - *continued*

Age-group	Sex	England and Wales (excluding port health authorities)	Wales	Standard regions							
				North	Yorkshire and Humberside	East Midlands	East Anglia	South East	South West	West Midlands	North West
Measles											
All ages	**M**	**7,005**	**301**	**796**	**928**	**505**	**187**	**1,833**	**481**	**875**	**1,099**
	F	**6,296**	**297**	**693**	**884**	**449**	**176**	**1,642**	**405**	**803**	**947**
Under 1 month	M	20	1	2	3	3	-	5	-	5	1
	F	16	1	1	-	3	-	6	2	1	2
1 month	M	19	-	2	7	-	-	4	-	3	3
	F	25	-	4	5	1	-	3	1	8	3
2 months	M	42	3	2	8	5	4	6	3	5	6
	F	35	1	2	4	2	-	8	1	10	7
3 months	M	51	3	2	10	2	2	15	1	8	8
	F	43	2	2	8	6	1	7	-	4	13
4 months	M	82	3	7	20	6	5	17	1	8	15
	F	61	3	4	9	6	3	17	3	8	8
5 months	M	89	2	12	9	7	1	27	4	8	19
	F	107	9	5	17	7	5	21	4	18	21
6 months	M	183	6	18	21	15	5	55	10	25	28
	F	154	7	8	24	22	7	34	10	19	23
7 months	M	157	8	11	22	12	2	40	8	28	26
	F	172	8	15	22	9	2	59	10	16	31
8 months	M	210	8	12	34	14	3	55	11	33	40
	F	211	15	11	27	22	7	53	17	22	37
9 months	M	221	15	14	23	15	3	70	15	31	35
	F	209	14	16	20	15	10	67	11	29	27
10 months	M	232	7	21	20	23	11	67	16	26	41
	F	202	8	13	26	9	5	67	17	20	37
11 months	M	218	10	18	17	16	5	74	14	26	38
	F	211	2	15	30	23	4	64	12	24	37
1 year	M	1,404	53	118	184	85	41	415	98	184	226
	F	1,367	47	113	193	105	48	371	99	173	218
2 years	M	597	15	53	100	37	20	159	31	74	108
	F	546	21	55	70	37	10	172	22	73	86
3 years	M	441	27	41	55	39	9	120	25	58	67
	F	396	27	46	40	23	12	95	29	67	57
4 years	M	446	23	59	60	28	9	100	23	67	77
	F	382	16	36	59	26	10	81	21	60	73
5 years	M	381	12	46	43	34	8	104	18	51	65
	F	336	21	37	49	28	5	91	14	46	45
6 years	M	293	11	51	38	26	7	71	13	27	49
	F	318	17	60	44	22	6	78	12	37	42
7 years	M	261	9	38	43	21	5	57	20	29	39
	F	238	14	34	38	12	6	62	12	27	33
8 years	M	198	8	44	18	15	8	38	20	21	26
	F	182	17	40	30	12	4	35	13	9	22
9 years	M	167	12	35	22	13	4	39	12	14	16
	F	182	4	40	35	6	7	35	15	21	19
10 - 14 years	M	476	18	96	62	26	19	94	62	39	60
	F	347	25	77	41	14	10	62	50	36	32
15 - 24 years	M	499	30	60	71	40	8	110	60	66	54
	F	224	9	28	42	11	8	54	16	30	26
25 and over	M	175	14	19	24	9	3	50	12	23	21
	F	187	5	21	29	19	3	47	10	28	25
Unknown	M	143	3	15	14	14	5	41	4	16	31
	F	145	4	10	22	9	3	53	4	17	23

Regional health authorities														Sex	Age-group
North-ern	York-shire	Trent	East Anglian	North West Thames	North East Thames	South East Thames	South West Thames	Wessex	Oxford	South West-ern	West Mid-lands	Mersey	North West-ern		
Measles															
796	**679**	**691**	**187**	**310**	**512**	**512**	**208**	**272**	**219**	**344**	**875**	**351**	**748**	M	**All ages**
693	**617**	**666**	**176**	**311**	**452**	**442**	**229**	**201**	**166**	**296**	**803**	**315**	**632**	F	
2	3	2	-	1	3	1	-	-	1	-	5	-	1	M	Under 1 month
1	-	3	-	1	1	1	1	1	1	2	1	-	2	F	
2	6	1	-	-	2	1	-	-	1	-	3	2	1	M	1 month
4	3	3	-	1	-	1	-	-	1	1	8	1	2	F	
2	7	5	4	-	2	2	-	2	2	2	5	3	3	M	2 months
2	2	4	-	4	1	2	-	-	1	1	10	5	2	F	
2	5	7	2	-	9	2	2	1	1	1	8	4	4	M	3 months
2	5	8	1	2	3	-	2	-	1	-	4	6	7	F	
7	10	15	5	3	8	-	4	-	3	1	8	4	11	M	4 months
4	5	10	3	4	4	4	-	3	2	3	8	1	7	F	
12	3	13	1	5	6	8	3	2	3	4	8	6	13	M	5 months
5	12	12	5	1	6	7	4	3	1	3	18	12	9	F	
18	16	19	5	15	17	11	7	6	4	6	25	9	19	M	6 months
8	18	26	7	3	6	12	9	7	2	7	19	12	11	F	
11	15	19	2	8	11	11	4	4	3	7	28	8	18	M	7 months
15	13	17	2	9	15	19	8	4	7	8	16	13	18	F	
12	25	23	3	7	19	14	6	5	6	9	33	12	28	M	8 months
11	20	26	7	12	20	13	5	7	4	12	22	9	28	F	
14	15	21	19	15	17	23	4	7	6	13	31	9	26	M	9 months
16	14	21	10	15	17	12	16	4	6	8	29	7	20	F	
21	13	27	11	10	16	24	9	10	6	11	26	16	25	M	10 months
13	22	9	5	9	24	10	12	7	13	13	20	12	25	F	
18	11	22	5	16	19	18	8	8	7	12	26	14	24	M	11 months
15	22	27	4	12	19	15	11	8	6	9	24	13	24	F	
118	154	100	41	68	116	132	44	46	50	72	184	69	157	M	1 year
113	140	146	48	67	104	104	48	52	38	69	173	74	144	F	
53	76	53	20	30	45	40	26	16	17	24	74	32	76	M	2 years
55	51	49	10	31	50	51	23	15	16	15	73	26	60	F	
41	35	56	9	18	30	39	13	16	14	18	58	18	49	M	3 years
46	30	32	12	24	22	23	14	14	6	22	67	18	39	F	
59	40	45	9	10	34	25	14	13	13	17	67	21	56	M	4 years
36	46	38	10	16	25	21	11	8	9	13	60	25	48	F	
46	32	42	8	20	27	31	13	10	9	15	51	24	41	M	5 years
37	32	43	5	17	27	20	14	7	10	12	46	12	33	F	
51	28	33	7	12	23	16	10	13	7	6	27	16	33	M	6 years
60	31	33	6	18	25	18	8	9	5	9	37	9	33	F	
38	33	28	5	11	20	17	2	14	6	10	29	17	22	M	7 years
34	22	28	6	11	11	23	7	5	7	10	27	13	20	F	
44	12	19	8	7	12	9	4	13	7	8	21	9	17	M	8 years
40	15	25	4	5	7	13	6	5	5	9	9	4	18	F	
35	19	14	4	3	8	11	4	9	10	8	14	4	12	M	9 years
40	26	14	7	7	6	9	7	6	3	13	21	6	13	F	
96	39	45	19	12	18	30	10	34	19	37	39	23	37	M	10 - 14 years
77	25	29	10	8	11	25	10	21	5	33	36	12	20	F	
60	54	52	8	19	25	21	11	33	17	49	66	19	35	M	15 - 24 years
28	25	27	8	7	18	13	7	4	7	15	30	14	12	F	
19	17	13	3	9	13	14	6	7	6	10	23	9	12	M	25 and over
21	20	25	3	12	13	12	4	6	6	7	28	9	16	F	
15	11	17	5	7	14	12	4	3	1	4	16	3	28	M	Unknown
10	18	11	3	15	17	14	2	5	4	2	17	2	21	F	

Table 4 Series MB2 no.17

Table 4 - *continued*

Age-group	Sex	England and Wales (excluding port health authorities)	Wales	Standard regions							
				North	Yorkshire and Humberside	East Midlands	East Anglia	South East	South West	West Midlands	North West
Rubella											
All ages	M	**6,298**	**213**	**532**	**1,191**	**558**	**198**	**1,511**	**569**	**663**	**863**
	F	**5,193**	**208**	**351**	**956**	**432**	**182**	**1,276**	**475**	**547**	**766**
Under 1 year	M	934	22	62	153	87	49	234	103	107	117
	F	881	22	54	123	90	39	238	93	90	132
1 year	M	821	19	55	125	78	27	226	98	92	101
	F	769	22	49	141	64	30	213	80	73	97
2 years	M	381	8	34	64	33	12	107	29	39	55
	F	358	18	24	69	31	14	107	30	27	38
3 years	M	399	15	35	75	30	9	95	29	41	70
	F	335	17	22	64	23	11	85	30	25	58
4 years	M	447	20	36	73	43	17	115	29	49	65
	F	374	17	25	65	38	10	94	20	47	58
5 years	M	396	17	36	80	37	14	87	24	44	57
	F	347	16	28	64	31	16	73	31	32	56
6 years	M	362	12	34	64	34	12	94	36	31	45
	F	369	21	18	77	21	14	85	35	40	58
7 years	M	276	11	28	61	16	13	57	25	29	36
	F	333	19	26	69	20	6	61	35	42	55
8 years	M	242	7	20	52	30	3	52	23	23	32
	F	289	10	21	58	24	15	61	29	31	40
9 years	M	251	19	19	43	28	6	49	24	27	36
	F	226	15	15	46	18	4	38	23	29	38
10-14 years	M	537	20	42	123	44	12	114	47	53	82
	F	354	12	32	61	26	8	74	32	46	63
15-24 year	M	881	29	103	210	72	14	181	74	90	108
	F	207	5	15	49	16	3	52	17	26	24
25 and over	M	270	11	23	48	18	9	74	22	25	40
	F	262	13	20	44	26	10	61	19	33	36
Unknown	M	101	3	5	20	8	1	26	6	13	19
	F	89	1	2	26	4	2	34	1	6	13
Acute encephalitis											
All ages	M	**21**	**1**	**-**	**6**	**1**	**-**	**9**	**1**	**1**	**2**
	F	**18**	**1**	**-**	**4**	**1**	**-**	**8**	**3**	**-**	**1**
Under 1 year	M	1	-	-	-	-	-	-	-	1	-
	F	2	-	-	-	-	-	2	-	-	-
1 year	M	-	-	-	-	-	-	-	-	-	-
	F	1	-	-	-	-	-	-	-	-	1
2 years	M	-	-	-	-	-	-	-	-	-	-
	F	1	-	-	-	-	-	1	-	-	-
3 years	M	1	-	-	-	-	-	1	-	-	-
	F	-	-	-	-	-	-	-	-	-	-
4 years	M	-	-	-	-	-	-	-	-	-	-
	F	1	-	-	1	-	-	-	-	-	-
5 - 9 years	M	4	-	-	1	1	-	1	-	-	1
	F	2	-	-	-	-	-	2	-	-	-
10 - 14 years	M	-	-	-	-	-	-	-	-	-	-
	F	2	-	-	-	-	-	2	-	-	-
15 - 24 years	M	3	-	-	1	-	-	1	1	-	-
	F	3	-	-	1	-	-	-	2	-	-
25 and over	M	12	1	-	4	-	-	6	-	-	1
	F	6	1	-	2	1	-	1	1	-	-
Unknown	M	-	-	-	-	-	-	-	-	-	-
	F	-	-	-	-	-	-	-	-	-	-

Regional health authorities														Sex	Age-group
North-ern	York-shire	Trent	East Anglian	North West Thames	North East Thames	South East Thames	South West Thames	Wessex	Oxford	South West-ern	West Mid-lands	Mersey	North West-ern		
Rubella															
532	**943**	**765**	**198**	**225**	**285**	**456**	**221**	**218**	**244**	**472**	**663**	**245**	**618**	M	All ages
351	**701**	**662**	**182**	**219**	**282**	**365**	**144**	**193**	**197**	**376**	**547**	**234**	**532**	F	
62	102	129	49	40	51	71	28	42	39	75	107	32	85	M	Under 1 year
54	86	122	39	35	59	61	27	42	44	68	90	23	109	F	
55	104	98	27	31	40	64	37	45	33	75	92	23	78	M	1 year
49	103	97	30	30	47	67	26	33	32	63	73	29	68	F	
34	48	46	12	15	27	30	21	8	13	25	39	14	41	M	2 years
24	57	42	14	20	29	31	11	13	11	23	27	10	28	F	
35	62	41	9	10	22	29	14	17	13	21	41	14	56	M	3 years
22	52	34	11	15	27	27	11	12	11	24	25	21	37	F	
36	56	56	17	18	27	33	14	11	18	27	49	16	49	M	4 years
25	50	50	10	20	19	27	12	8	15	16	47	14	44	F	
36	59	56	14	15	19	25	9	13	14	18	44	19	38	M	5 years
28	41	51	16	17	21	19	5	11	10	24	32	20	36	F	
34	56	42	12	18	18	25	14	8	14	33	31	9	36	M	6 years
18	55	41	14	19	13	27	7	16	13	27	40	16	42	F	
28	40	37	13	7	6	22	9	13	6	19	29	14	22	M	7 years
26	49	39	6	7	15	19	4	13	9	30	42	20	35	F	
20	34	45	3	10	9	14	3	7	14	21	23	10	22	M	8 years
21	49	31	15	11	12	17	5	8	13	26	31	16	24	F	
19	29	40	6	6	11	10	9	6	11	22	27	13	23	M	9 years
15	27	37	4	10	2	7	4	11	8	19	29	16	22	F	
42	96	67	12	14	13	50	13	12	22	41	53	33	49	M	10-14 years
32	43	43	8	11	18	21	9	12	10	26	46	26	37	F	
103	200	74	14	27	27	50	30	29	31	69	90	28	80	M	15-24 years
15	34	31	3	10	12	14	7	4	6	16	26	5	19	F	
23	42	21	9	11	8	23	18	6	13	20	25	16	24	M	25 and over
20	33	36	10	6	13	16	11	9	12	14	33	15	21	F	
5	15	13	1	3	7	10	2	1	3	6	13	4	15	M	Unknown
2	22	8	2	7	7	12	5	1	3	-	6	3	10	F	
Acute Encephalitis															
.	.	6	.	2	3	2	1	1	1	1	1	1	1	M	All ages
.	1	4	.	4	2	1	-	1	1	2	-	-	1	F	
-	-	-	-	-	-	-	-	-	-	-	1	-	-	M	Under 1 year
-	-	-	-	1	-	-	-	-	1	-	-	-	-	F	
-	-	-	-	-	-	-	-	-	-	-	-	-	-	M	1 year
-	-	-	-	-	-	-	-	-	-	-	-	-	1	F	
-	-	-	-	-	-	-	-	-	-	-	-	-	-	M	2 years
-	-	-	-	-	-	1	-	-	-	-	-	-	-	F	
-	-	-	-	-	-	1	-	-	-	-	-	-	-	M	3 years
-	-	-	-	-	-	-	-	-	-	-	-	-	-	F	
-	-	-	-	-	-	-	-	-	-	-	-	-	-	M	4 years
-	1	-	-	-	-	-	-	-	-	-	-	-	-	F	
-	-	1	-	-	1	-	-	-	1	-	-	1	-	M	5-9 years
-	-	-	-	1	1	-	-	-	-	-	-	-	-	F	
-	-	-	-	-	-	-	-	-	-	-	-	-	-	M	10-14 years
-	-	-	-	2	-	-	-	-	-	-	-	-	-	F	
-	-	1	-	1	-	-	-	-	-	1	-	-	-	M	15-24 years
-	-	1	-	-	-	-	-	1	-	1	-	-	-	F	
-	-	4	-	1	2	1	1	1	-	-	-	-	1	M	25 and over
-	-	3	-	-	1	-	-	-	-	1	-	-	-	F	
-	-	-	-	-	-	-	-	-	-	-	-	-	-	M	Unknown
-	-	-	-	-	-	-	-	-	-	-	-	-	-	F	

Table 4 Series MB2 no.17

Table 4 - *continued*

Age-group	Sex	England and Wales (excluding port health authorities)	Wales	Standard regions							
				North	Yorkshire and Humberside	East Midlands	East Anglia	South East	South West	West Midlands	North West
Viral hepatitis											
All ages	M	**4,770**	**130**	**612**	**915**	**283**	**81**	**1,336**	**277**	**304**	**832**
	F	**4,235**	**127**	**620**	**863**	**258**	**52**	**1,103**	**231**	**266**	**715**
Under 1 year	M	9	1	3	1	-	-	4	-	-	-
	F	6	-	1	1	1	-	1	-	-	2
1 year	M	23	-	4	7	-	-	4	1	-	7
	F	10	-	2	6	-	-	-	-	1	1
2-4 years	M	217	9	33	55	5	3	41	6	12	53
	F	208	12	33	60	13	1	34	8	10	37
5-9 years	M	906	20	141	213	53	7	186	38	50	198
	F	923	34	172	194	52	6	186	44	48	187
10-14 years	M	654	17	108	150	38	9	125	29	55	123
	F	604	8	119	133	41	8	112	32	35	116
15-19 years	M	475	7	73	100	35	8	106	21	35	90
	F	366	9	61	78	20	5	84	17	27	65
20-24 years	M	515	17	65	86	31	7	150	32	38	89
	F	415	13	50	78	28	7	103	29	29	78
25-34 years	M	951	28	104	142	59	17	354	55	53	139
	F	849	28	122	149	51	12	271	49	46	121
35-44 years	M	489	11	39	68	30	20	179	50	26	66
	F	422	7	36	88	24	4	159	31	31	42
45-54 years	M	237	7	17	36	19	5	90	23	15	25
	F	163	2	12	26	10	2	59	10	15	27
55-64 years	M	105	6	11	18	2	1	39	11	6	11
	F	93	3	6	16	7	-	37	5	10	9
65-74 years	M	58	2	5	15	5	-	18	6	5	2
	F	50	1	1	9	6	4	19	4	4	2
75 and over	M	29	1	5	2	2	1	11	1	3	3
	F	27	-	-	4	2	1	10	2	3	5
Unknown	M	102	4	4	22	4	3	29	4	6	26
	F	99	10	5	21	3	2	28	-	7	23
Mumps											
All ages	M	**2,330**	**124**	**115**	**253**	**213**	**115**	**611**	**240**	**317**	**342**
	F	**1,947**	**95**	**113**	**250**	**150**	**82**	**550**	**202**	**251**	**254**
Under 1 year	M	48	2	-	6	5	-	16	4	6	9
	F	29	2	1	1	2	-	15	2	4	2
1 year	M	195	4	7	19	18	6	53	23	27	38
	F	96	4	3	10	2	4	30	15	9	19
2 years	M	169	8	11	17	19	11	43	18	17	25
	F	125	2	7	22	11	6	30	17	12	18
3 years	M	265	12	15	25	25	10	75	25	34	44
	F	152	3	10	17	9	4	51	9	22	27
4 years	M	307	18	16	34	37	11	82	33	32	44
	F	230	12	11	33	23	8	56	25	27	35
5 years	M	221	13	14	34	23	12	45	18	32	30
	F	166	11	11	20	17	9	42	17	19	20
6 years	M	173	13	8	13	12	7	46	20	28	26
	F	159	8	11	20	11	11	37	18	23	20
7 years	M	146	9	4	14	6	9	38	14	27	25
	F	108	7	7	12	14	4	23	10	18	13
8 years	M	114	8	7	15	8	4	26	11	14	21
	F	97	4	5	14	3	1	32	13	10	15
9 years	M	87	9	5	8	7	7	21	6	15	9
	F	86	7	5	10	7	1	23	13	10	10
10-14 years	M	216	9	15	28	15	9	65	27	29	19
	F	221	11	16	28	17	10	65	24	24	26
15-24 years	M	110	5	2	12	6	12	28	14	17	14
	F	178	12	11	18	13	11	50	19	21	23
25 and over	M	243	12	10	20	28	16	60	24	38	35
	F	275	10	14	42	21	13	82	18	50	25
Unknown	M	36	2	1	8	4	1	13	3	1	3
	F	25	2	1	3	-	-	14	2	2	1

Northern	Yorkshire	Trent	East Anglian	North West Thames	North East Thames	South East Thames	South West Thames	Wessex	Oxford	South Western	West Midlands	Mersey	North Western	Sex	Age-group
Regional health authorities														Sex	Age-group
Viral hepatitis															
612	**808**	**273**	**81**	**172**	**248**	**484**	**140**	**115**	**366**	**205**	**304**	**281**	**551**	M	All ages
620	**777**	**214**	**52**	**131**	**179**	**453**	**102**	**59**	**346**	**194**	**266**	**222**	**493**	F	
3	1	-	-	-	3	-	-	-	1	-	-	-	-	M	Under 1 year
1	1	1	-	-	-	-	-	-	1	-	-	2	-	F	
4	7	-	-	-	-	2	-	-	2	1	-	6	1	M	1 year
2	5	1	-	-	-	-	-	-	-	-	1	-	1	F	
33	49	7	3	4	6	23	2	-	10	6	12	31	22	M	2-4 years
33	60	6	1	4	7	16	2	1	11	8	10	18	19	F	
141	198	34	7	25	28	77	12	8	75	33	50	76	122	M	5-9 years
172	177	29	6	29	19	84	13	4	81	40	48	61	126	F	
108	134	29	9	12	27	46	6	9	56	23	55	38	85	M	10-14 years
119	119	28	8	18	19	36	16	8	48	26	35	38	78	F	
73	93	33	8	13	14	44	11	12	25	17	35	22	68	M	15-19 years
61	72	18	5	9	15	35	8	4	24	14	27	21	44	F	
65	71	39	7	19	32	48	15	22	35	18	38	28	61	M	20-24 years
50	65	28	7	10	16	50	7	6	31	25	29	24	54	F	
104	118	61	17	47	68	136	38	22	75	45	53	38	101	M	25-34 years
122	133	52	12	30	50	123	16	14	61	41	46	36	85	F	
39	51	42	20	28	29	55	33	17	38	34	26	18	48	M	35-44 years
36	76	25	4	16	28	55	19	12	48	23	31	8	34	F	
17	34	15	5	14	13	30	9	15	25	13	15	11	14	M	45-54 years
12	23	10	2	5	9	19	13	3	14	9	15	7	20	F	
11	16	3	1	4	13	5	4	5	12	8	6	5	6	M	55-64 years
6	14	7	-	3	5	12	5	1	13	5	10	3	6	F	
5	14	4	-	1	3	5	5	4	5	3	5	1	1	M	65-74 years
1	9	3	4	3	3	8	-	3	7	2	4	-	2	F	
5	2	2	1	2	4	-	-	1	5	-	3	1	2	M	75 and over
-	4	1	1	1	1	3	1	1	5	1	3	2	3	F	
4	20	4	3	3	8	13	5	-	2	4	6	6	20	M	Unknown
5	19	5	2	3	7	12	2	2	2	-	7	2	21	F	
Mumps															
115	**199**	**242**	**115**	**107**	**122**	**152**	**72**	**156**	**103**	**164**	**317**	**119**	**223**	M	All ages
113	**172**	**213**	**82**	**83**	**126**	**132**	**71**	**119**	**90**	**146**	**251**	**73**	**181**	F	
-	6	5	-	2	3	5	4	4	1	1	6	7	2	M	Under 1 year
1	1	2	-	4	4	2	1	3	3	-	4	1	1	F	
7	13	23	6	9	12	9	9	11	10	17	27	19	19	M	1 year
3	6	6	4	6	6	6	2	7	7	11	9	7	12	F	
11	12	19	11	11	12	12	4	7	7	13	17	9	16	M	2 years
7	17	16	6	4	8	8	2	9	2	14	12	4	14	F	
15	19	28	10	9	18	17	6	22	15	16	34	13	31	M	3 years
10	10	14	4	5	15	13	4	6	14	5	22	9	18	F	
16	27	41	11	11	20	21	9	21	13	23	32	16	28	M	4 years
11	25	29	8	6	11	12	7	16	14	17	27	12	23	F	
14	26	30	12	9	5	14	5	11	6	14	32	11	19	M	5 years
11	9	27	9	8	12	10	3	10	5	12	19	5	15	F	
8	11	12	7	9	9	12	4	17	6	11	28	8	18	M	6 years
11	15	16	11	4	10	9	7	13	3	9	23	6	14	F	
4	12	7	9	6	6	8	6	12	4	11	27	5	20	M	7 years
7	10	16	4	2	5	9	3	5	1	8	18	4	9	F	
7	13	9	4	8	5	6	2	7	2	8	14	8	13	M	8 years
5	9	7	1	10	6	8	3	7	1	11	10	2	13	F	
5	8	6	7	2	3	6	1	7	7	2	15	4	5	M	9 years
5	7	10	1	3	4	6	2	7	5	9	10	-	10	F	
15	21	21	9	15	9	21	5	10	13	20	29	7	12	M	10-14 years
16	18	22	10	12	9	19	8	11	16	19	24	9	17	F	
2	8	9	12	4	5	2	4	10	7	11	17	2	12	M	15-24 years
11	12	18	11	4	14	11	10	12	5	14	21	7	16	F	
10	16	27	16	10	12	14	10	17	12	14	38	10	25	M	25 and over
14	31	29	13	14	19	16	14	11	14	15	50	7	18	F	
1	7	5	1	2	3	5	3	-	-	3	1	-	3	M	Unknown
1	2	1	-	1	3	3	5	2	-	2	2	-	1	F	

Table 4 Series MB2 no.17

Table 4 - *continued*

Age-group	Sex	England and Wales (excluding port health authorities)	Wales	Standard regions							
				North	Yorkshire and Humberside	East Midlands	East Anglia	South East	South West	West Midlands	North West
Malaria											
All ages	M	**937**	**20**	**15**	**96**	**62**	**16**	**544**	**40**	**87**	**57**
	F	**556**	**4**	**6**	**44**	**54**	**6**	**328**	**16**	**61**	**37**
0 - 4 years	M	32	-	-	9	4	1	9	-	5	4
	F	19	-	-	3	2	1	9	-	-	4
5 - 14 years	M	93	1	-	19	6	1	46	2	8	10
	F	73	1	1	8	5	1	34	3	11	9
15 - 24 years	M	184	8	3	20	5	5	117	9	10	7
	F	125	1	2	5	11	2	84	3	10	7
25 - 44 years	M	408	6	5	26	27	6	264	20	29	25
	F	196	2	2	16	18	1	130	4	14	9
45 - 64 years	M	151	4	4	14	10	2	81	7	22	7
	F	108	-	1	9	13	1	51	6	20	7
65 and over	M	48	-	3	7	10	1	15	2	9	1
	F	24	-	-	3	5	-	11	-	4	1
Unknown	M	21	1	-	1	-	-	12	-	4	3
	F	11	-	-	-	-	-	9	-	2	-
Leptospirosis											
All ages	M	**18**	**-**	**1**	**3**	**1**	**3**	**4**	**1**	**2**	**3**
	F	**2**	**1**	**-**	**-**	**-**	**-**	**-**	**1**	**-**	**-**
0 - 4 years	M	-	-	-	-	-	-	-	-	-	-
	F	-	-	-	-	-	-	-	-	-	-
5 - 14 years	M	-	-	-	-	-	-	-	-	-	-
	F	-	-	-	-	-	-	-	-	-	-
15 - 24 years	M	-	-	-	-	-	-	-	-	-	-
	F	-	-	-	-	-	-	-	-	-	-
25 - 44 years	M	13	-	-	3	1	2	2	-	2	3
	F	1	-	-	-	-	-	-	1	-	-
45 - 64 years	M	5	-	1	-	-	1	2	1	-	-
	F	1	1	-	-	-	-	-	-	-	-
65 and over	M	-	-	-	-	-	-	-	-	-	-
	F	-	-	-	-	-	-	-	-	-	-
Unknown	M	-	-	-	-	-	-	-	-	-	-
	F	-	-	-	-	-	-	-	-	-	-
Tetanus											
All ages	M	**3**	**-**	**1**	**-**	**-**	**-**	**-**	**2**	**-**	**-**
	F	**6**	**-**	**-**	**-**	**-**	**-**	**5**	**-**	**-**	**1**
0 - 4 years	M	-	-	-	-	-	-	-	-	-	-
	F	-	-	-	-	-	-	-	-	-	-
5 - 14 years	M	-	-	-	-	-	-	-	-	-	-
	F	-	-	-	-	-	-	-	-	-	-
15 - 24 years	M	-	-	-	-	-	-	-	-	-	-
	F	1	-	-	-	-	-	1	-	-	-
25 - 44 years	M	-	-	-	-	-	-	-	-	-	-
	F	-	-	-	-	-	-	-	-	-	-
45 - 64 years	M	1	-	1	-	-	-	-	-	-	-
	F	1	-	-	-	-	-	-	-	-	1
65 and over	M	2	-	-	-	-	-	-	2	-	-
	F	4	-	-	-	-	-	4	-	-	-
Unknown	M	-	-	-	-	-	-	-	-	-	-
	F	-	-	-	-	-	-	-	-	-	-
Ophthalmia neonatorum											
All ages	M	**252**	**8**	**8**	**27**	**18**	**2**	**75**	**14**	**50**	**50**
	F	**188**	**4**	**3**	**24**	**13**	**1**	**59**	**10**	**36**	**38**
Acute Poliomyelitis (paralytic)											
All ages	M	**1**	**-**	**-**	**-**	**-**	**-**	**-**	**-**	**-**	**1**
	F	**-**	**-**	**-**	**-**	**-**	**-**	**-**	**-**	**-**	**-**
Under 1 year	M	1	-	-	-	-	-	-	-	-	1
	F	-	-	-	-	-	-	-	-	-	-

Regional health authorities

Malaria

North-ern	York-shire	Trent	East Anglian	North West Thames	North East Thames	South East Thames	South West Thames	Wessex	Oxford	South West-ern	West Mid-lands	Mersey	North West-ern	Sex	Age-group
15	76	77	16	205	141	83	75	24	33	28	87	10	47	M	All ages
6	36	55	6	133	91	44	38	9	25	11	61	5	32	F	
-	9	4	1	4	1	1	2	-	1	-	5	-	4	M	0 - 4 years
-	3	1	1	2	3	1	2	-	2	-	-	-	4	F	
-	16	9	1	27	6	7	6	-	-	2	8	1	9	M	5 - 14 years
1	8	4	1	17	7	4	4	2	3	1	11	-	9	F	
3	15	10	5	43	33	17	16	5	6	6	10	1	6	M	15 - 24 years
2	3	12	2	26	25	13	13	2	8	1	10	3	4	F	
5	17	32	6	82	81	46	34	12	19	14	29	7	18	M	25 - 44 years
2	13	17	1	55	41	19	7	2	10	4	14	1	8	F	
4	12	11	2	33	14	9	16	6	6	5	22	1	6	M	45 - 64 years
1	7	15	1	24	9	6	8	3	2	5	20	1	6	F	
3	6	11	1	10	3	1	1	1	-	1	9	-	1	M	65 and over
-	2	6	-	6	2	1	2	-	-	-	4	-	1	F	
-	1	-	-	6	3	2	-	-	1	-	4	-	3	M	Unknown
-	-	-	-	3	4	-	2	-	-	-	2	-	-	F	

Leptospirosis

North-ern	York-shire	Trent	East Anglian	North West Thames	North East Thames	South East Thames	South West Thames	Wessex	Oxford	South West-ern	West Mid-lands	Mersey	North West-ern	Sex	Age-group
1	3	1	3	-	-	3	-	-	1	1	2	3	-	M	All ages
-	-	-	-	-	-	-	-	-	-	1	-	-	-	F	
-	-	-	-	-	-	-	-	-	-	-	-	-	-	M	0 - 4 years
-	-	-	-	-	-	-	-	-	-	-	-	-	-	F	
-	-	-	-	-	-	-	-	-	-	-	-	-	-	M	5 - 14 years
-	-	-	-	-	-	-	-	-	-	-	-	-	-	F	
-	-	-	-	-	-	-	-	-	-	-	-	-	-	M	15 - 24 years
-	-	-	-	-	-	-	-	-	-	-	-	-	-	F	
-	3	1	2	-	-	2	-	-	-	-	2	3	-	M	25 - 44 years
-	-	-	-	-	-	-	-	-	-	1	-	-	-	F	
1	-	-	1	-	-	1	-	-	1	1	-	-	-	M	45 - 64 years
-	-	-	-	-	-	-	-	-	-	-	-	-	-	F	
-	-	-	-	-	-	-	-	-	-	-	-	-	-	M	65 and over
-	-	-	-	-	-	-	-	-	-	-	-	-	-	F	
-	-	-	-	-	-	-	-	-	-	-	-	-	-	M	Unknown
-	-	-	-	-	-	-	-	-	-	-	-	-	-	F	

Tetanus

North-ern	York-shire	Trent	East Anglian	North West Thames	North East Thames	South East Thames	South West Thames	Wessex	Oxford	South West-ern	West Mid-lands	Mersey	North West-ern	Sex	Age-group
1	-	-	-	-	-	-	-	-	-	2	-	-	-	M	All ages
-	-	-	-	-	-	3	1	-	1	-	-	1	-	F	
-	-	-	-	-	-	-	-	-	-	-	-	-	-	M	0 - 4 years
-	-	-	-	-	-	-	-	-	-	-	-	-	-	F	
-	-	-	-	-	-	-	-	-	-	-	-	-	-	M	5 - 14 years
-	-	-	-	-	-	-	-	-	-	-	-	-	-	F	
-	-	-	-	-	-	1	-	-	-	-	-	-	-	M	15 - 24 years
-	-	-	-	-	-	-	-	-	-	-	-	-	-	F	
-	-	-	-	-	-	-	-	-	-	-	-	-	-	M	25 - 44 years
-	-	-	-	-	-	-	-	-	-	-	-	-	-	F	
1	-	-	-	-	-	-	-	-	-	-	-	-	-	M	45 - 64 years
-	-	-	-	-	-	-	-	-	-	-	-	1	-	F	
-	-	-	-	-	-	-	-	-	-	2	-	-	-	M	65 and over
-	-	-	-	-	-	2	1	-	1	-	-	-	-	F	
-	-	-	-	-	-	-	-	-	-	-	-	-	-	M	Unknown
-	-	-	-	-	-	-	-	-	-	-	-	-	-	F	

Ophthalmia neonatorum

North-ern	York-shire	Trent	East Anglian	North West Thames	North East Thames	South East Thames	South West Thames	Wessex	Oxford	South West-ern	West Mid-lands	Mersey	North West-ern	Sex	Age-group
8	20	24	2	11	17	13	5	10	23	11	50	19	31	M	All ages
3	22	15	1	6	12	23	2	3	14	9	36	16	22	F	

Acute Poliomyelitis (paralytic)

North-ern	York-shire	Trent	East Anglian	North West Thames	North East Thames	South East Thames	South West Thames	Wessex	Oxford	South West-ern	West Mid-lands	Mersey	North West-ern	Sex	Age-group
-	-	-	-	-	-	-	-	-	-	-	-	-	1	M	All ages
-	-	-	-	-	-	-	-	-	-	-	-	-	-	F	
-	-	-	-	-	-	-	-	-	-	-	-	-	1	M	Under 1 year
-	-	-	-	-	-	-	-	-	-	-	-	-	-	F	

Table 5 Series MB2 no.17

Table 5 Corrected notifications of selected infectious diseases, 1990

England and Wales, standard regions, regional health authorities, Greater London, London boroughs, metropolitan and non-metropolitan counties and districts, port health authorities

Area	Typhoid fever	Paratyphoid fever	Dysentery (amoebic and bacillary)	Food poisoning — Formally notified	Food poisoning — Ascertained by other means	Tuberculosis — All tuberculosis≠	All respiratory TB†	All pulmonary TB†	All TB meningitis†	Other forms of TB†	Whooping cough	Scarlet fever	Meningitis — All meningitis	Meningococcal meningitis	Meningococcal septicaemia (without meningitis)	Measles	Rubella	Viral hepatitis	Mumps	Malaria
England & Wales (excluding port health authorities)	177	93	2,756	36,945	15,200	5,204	3,942	3,618	81	1,228	15,286	7,187	2,572	1,138	277	13,301	11,491	9,005	4,277	1,493
Wales	1	1	235	2,528	495	194	163	152	4	27	1,161	199	203	71	22	598	421	257	219	24
Standard regions																				
North	2	3	48	2,881	1,047	205	170	146	2	33	1,530	438	146	76	19	1,489	883	1,232	228	21
Yorkshire and Humberside	29	13	552	5,002	2,166	537	398	372	5	143	2,029	1,360	344	136	33	1,812	2,147	1,778	503	140
East Midlands	10	4	127	3,131	906	404	331	272	8	67	936	603	163	77	18	954	990	541	363	116
East Anglia	1	3	47	1,164	254	97	73	71	3	22	508	186	76	34	6	363	380	133	197	22
South East	93	35	995	12,320	4,160	2,119	1,589	1,446	37	511	3,983	2,198	727	317	77	3,475	2,787	2,439	1,161	872
of which																				
Greater London	71	24	482	4,469	966	1,603	1,225	1,103	10	378	1,232	765	292	133	36	1,371	936	767	409	693
South West	2	4	248	3,282	1,842	173	140	129	3	31	1,281	595	232	100	22	886	1,044	508	442	56
West Midlands	23	16	198	2,831	2,548	732	511	488	10	224	1,457	824	262	116	23	1,678	1,210	570	568	148
North West	16	14	306	3,806	1,782	743	567	542	9	170	2,401	784	419	211	57	2,046	1,629	1,547	596	94
Regional health authorities																				
Northern	2	3	48	2,881	1,047	205	170	146	2	33	1,530	438	146	76	19	1,489	883	1,232	228	21
Yorkshire	24	13	519	3,920	1,721	437	321	295	5	118	1,582	1,035	254	100	26	1,296	1,644	1,585	371	112
Trent	13	4	145	3,621	1,247	452	366	310	7	83	1,249	866	222	104	21	1,357	1,427	487	455	132
East Anglian	1	3	47	1,164	254	97	73	71	3	22	508	186	76	34	6	363	380	133	197	22
North West Thames	40	13	297	2,507	731	645	465	430	3	184	725	393	139	67	17	621	444	303	190	338
North East Thames	25	12	209	2,756	775	670	530	449	10	135	920	542	168	66	17	964	567	427	248	232
South East Thames	10	2	131	2,502	780	382	296	280	6	81	969	525	168	71	9	954	821	937	284	127
South West Thames	12	4	177	2,160	913	258	187	182	4	70	593	350	105	46	12	437	365	242	143	113
Wessex	-	1	85	1,568	1,147	111	84	78	1	27	676	351	107	49	7	473	411	174	275	33
Oxford	8	4	171	2,191	488	164	117	114	15	34	553	298	115	42	20	385	441	712	193	58
South Western	2	3	188	2,510	1,272	114	92	81	2	20	962	396	188	85	21	640	848	399	310	39
West Midlands	23	16	198	2,831	2,548	732	511	488	10	224	1,457	824	262	116	23	1,678	1,210	570	568	148
Mersey	1	2	35	1,670	143	139	113	110	-	27	948	378	162	78	28	666	479	503	192	15
North Western	15	12	271	2,136	1,639	604	454	432	9	143	1,453	406	257	133	29	1,380	1,150	1,044	404	79
Northern RHA																				
Tyne and Wear*	2	2	14	691	467	104	84	77	1	19	590	83	69	43	9	826	315	502	60	9
Gateshead	-	-	4	44	406	16	12	12	-	4	105	10	18	14	1	123	37	175	3	-
Newcastle upon Tyne	1	-	4	86	1	36	26	23	-	10	115	11	14	11	3	70	84	175	8	5
North Tyneside	-	-	4	224	60	19	17	13	1	1	60	4	10	4	4	49	37	94	3	1
South Tyneside	1	-	-	151	-	4	4	4	-	-	102	14	10	3	1	364	21	25	8	2
Sunderland	-	2	2	186	-	29	25	25	-	4	208	44	17	11	-	220	136	33	38	1
Cleveland	-	-	6	415	120	42	40	24	-	2	242	105	25	10	1	122	163	492	35	4
Hartlepool	-	-	-	11	41	8	7	7	-	1	22	12	8	1	-	20	12	318	1	-
Langbaurgh-on-Tees	-	-	-	105	-	8	8	3	-	-	67	8	7	2	-	28	28	19	7	-
Middlesbrough	-	-	4	119	72	17	17	9	-	-	58	38	2	2	1	20	47	13	7	4
Stockton-on-Tees	-	-	2	180	7	9	8	5	-	1	95	47	8	5	-	54	76	142	20	-
Cumbria	-	1	6	1,013	217	23	17	17	-	6	181	62	21	8	4	73	39	40	22	4
Allerdale	-	-	-	324	-	5	5	5	-	-	66	18	5	2	2	5	8	2	2	-
Barrow-in-Furness	-	-	-	55	-	-	-	-	-	-	13	1	-	-	-	12	1	-	3	-
Carlisle	-	-	3	27	152	8	5	5	-	3	14	14	8	2	-	19	10	18	2	1
Copeland	-	1	-	231	-	4	4	4	-	-	54	26	2	1	1	10	13	3	10	1
Eden	-	-	2	22	64	3	1	1	-	2	13	1	5	3	1	2	-	9	3	-
South Lakeland	-	-	1	354	1	3	2	2	-	1	21	2	1	-	-	25	7	8	2	2
Durham	-	-	17	636	198	28	22	21	-	6	410	181	28	14	3	381	298	156	83	3
Chester-le-Street	-	-	6	25	-	2	1	-	-	1	51	58	3	2	-	14	6	4	6	-
Darlington	-	-	2	102	106	4	4	4	-	-	56	15	7	3	3	69	44	22	4	-
Derwentside	-	-	3	90	10	8	7	7	-	1	29	28	4	3	-	77	31	50	5	-
Durham	-	-	1	69	8	7	7	7	-	-	69	38	6	3	-	53	36	3	32	3
Easington	-	-	2	36	-	2	1	1	-	1	46	3	2	-	-	22	38	12	11	-
Sedgefield	-	-	3	127	-	3	2	2	-	1	55	23	2	1	-	55	95	11	11	-
Teesdale	-	-	-	42	-	-	-	-	-	-	6	12	1	1	-	14	18	1	8	-
Wear Valley	-	-	-	145	74	2	-	-	-	2	98	4	3	1	-	77	30	53	6	-

See note on page viii.

* Metropolitan county.

† Categories overlap and therefore some cases will be included in more than one column.

≠ See note on page vi.

Table 5 - *continued*

Area	Typhoid fever	Paratyphoid fever	Dysentery (amoebic and bacillary)	Food poisoning Formally notified	Food poisoning Ascertained by other means	Tuberculosis All tuberculosis≠	All respiratory TB†	All pulmonary TB†	All TB meningitis†	Other forms of TB†	Whooping cough	Scarlet fever	All meningitis	Meningococcal meningitis	Meningococcal septicaemia (without meningitis)	Measles	Rubella	Viral hepatitis	Mumps	Malaria
Northern RHA - *continued*																				
Northumberland	-	-	5	126	45	8	7	7	1	-	107	7	3	1	2	87	68	42	28	1
Alnwick	-	-	3	9	15	-	-	-	-	-	4	-	-	-	1	7	4	-	9	-
Berwick-upon-Tweed	-	-	-	5	2	1	1	1	-	-	3	-	-	-	-	5	7	15	1	-
Blyth Valley	-	-	-	21	4	3	2	2	1	-	7	1	1	-	-	46	16	6	7	-
Castle Morpeth	-	-	-	17	9	2	2	2	-	-	33	2	-	-	-	13	10	4	4	1
Tynedale	-	-	2	51	9	-	-	-	-	-	15	2	2	1	1	5	2	10	2	-
Wansbeck	-	-	-	23	6	2	2	2	-	-	45	2	-	-	-	11	29	7	5	-
Yorkshire RHA																				
West Yorkshire*	21	11	459	2,457	1,298	379	273	251	5	108	921	541	137	49	18	813	940	1,340	215	92
Bradford	14	7	67	676	363	150	97	93	2	54	109	100	35	13	6	171	120	464	32	45
Calderdale	2	2	14	30	64	35	26	25	-	9	95	52	10	9	-	88	84	349	14	5
Kirklees	4	-	83	606	129	99	72	55	1	26	193	88	20	8	4	141	59	200	56	22
Leeds	1	2	288	962	628	78	67	67	1	13	415	195	43	12	6	244	526	277	74	18
Wakefield	-	-	7	183	114	17	11	11	1	6	109	106	29	7	2	169	151	50	39	2
Humberside	-	2	36	787	174	34	29	25	-	5	314	183	74	32	8	350	453	142	93	7
Boothferry	-	-	-	48	7	-	-	-	-	-	13	6	4	-	1	23	13	6	5	-
Cleethorpes	-	-	12	237	60	5	3	3	-	2	20	26	3	2	1	24	20	-	3	2
East Yorkshire	-	-	-	32	-	5	5	4	-	-	35	38	9	6	-	12	48	2	10	-
E Yorks Boro of Beverley	-	1	1	67	2	4	4	4	-	-	18	19	12	2	-	10	16	34	8	1
Glanford	-	-	2	26	29	3	3	3	-	-	37	-	-	-	-	20	39	10	6	-
Great Grimsby	-	-	6	301	2	3	3	3	-	-	42	46	10	8	1	66	36	2	14	-
Holderness	-	-	1	-	-	-	-	-	-	-	9	18	6	3	-	37	62	1	5	-
Kingston upon Hull	-	1	12	12	41	10	7	5	-	3	123	30	29	11	5	106	131	80	32	4
Scunthorpe	-	-	2	64	33	4	4	3	-	-	17	-	1	-	-	52	88	7	10	-
North Yorkshire	3	-	24	676	249	24	19	19	-	5	347	311	43	19	-	133	251	103	63	13
Craven	1	-	3	31	13	1	1	1	-	-	43	9	3	-	-	3	1	22	-	1
Hambleton	-	-	1	51	-	3	3	3	-	-	30	4	5	2	-	18	11	14	7	-
Harrogate	-	-	9	228	204	5	5	5	-	-	75	55	5	2	-	40	133	22	10	2
Richmondshire	2	-	-	42	31	1	-	-	-	1	9	30	3	2	-	13	23	4	6	5
Ryedale	-	-	1	87	-	2	2	2	-	-	26	35	2	-	-	16	9	7	7	-
Scarborough	-	-	4	93	-	7	4	4	-	3	53	147	6	1	-	15	44	16	24	-
Selby	-	-	3	48	-	3	3	3	-	-	89	9	11	9	-	11	13	5	4	-
York	-	-	3	96	1	2	1	1	-	1	22	22	8	3	-	17	17	13	5	5
Trent RHA																				
South Yorkshire*	5	-	33	1,082	445	100	77	77	-	25	447	325	90	36	7	516	503	193	132	28
Barnsley	-	-	1	30	-	13	9	9	-	4	108	36	11	3	-	65	47	7	12	-
Doncaster	-	-	4	72	134	18	14	14	-	4	61	47	20	13	2	150	165	96	36	2
Rotherham	-	-	5	180	47	21	14	14	-	8	130	125	24	9	2	136	141	39	34	2
Sheffield	5	-	23	800	264	48	40	40	-	9	148	117	35	11	3	165	150	51	50	24
Derbyshire	2	-	12	663	44	61	37	36	3	21	238	162	41	23	6	259	178	38	77	14
Amber Valley	-	-	-	47	-	2	1	1	-	1	36	6	7	4	1	13	25	1	4	-
Bolsover	-	-	1	27	7	1	1	1	-	-	8	2	1	-	-	15	5	8	3	-
Chesterfield	-	-	-	129	-	2	1	1	-	1	16	23	3	2	2	33	21	-	7	-
Derby	1	-	8	138	13	42	25	24	1	16	70	43	16	10	1	77	34	10	26	13
Derbyshire Dales	-	-	2	64	1	1	1	1	-	-	18	5	2	1	1	11	7	1	4	-
Erewash	-	-	1	60	-	9	5	5	2	2	16	14	3	2	-	41	32	5	5	-
High Peak**	1	-	-	94	-	2	2	2	-	-	14	8	3	1	-	38	26	7	18	-
North East Derbyshire	-	-	-	92	23	1	-	-	-	1	20	42	2	1	1	3	4	5	4	-
South Derbyshire	-	-	-	12	-	1	1	1	-	-	40	19	4	2	-	28	24	1	6	1
Leicestershire	5	3	30	632	122	186	171	116	3	12	201	131	20	9	-	272	391	64	100	73
Blaby	-	-	1	60	-	1	1	1	-	-	16	5	1	-	-	10	49	12	6	1
Charnwood	-	-	2	64	-	14	13	12	1	-	49	13	4	3	-	36	90	7	20	-
Harborough	-	-	3	232	1	1	1	-	-	-	8	18	-	-	-	22	23	6	8	1
Hinckley & Bosworth	-	-	-	111	12	6	1	1	1	4	19	43	2	-	-	58	33	7	3	-
Leicester	5	3	18	38	89	152	147	95	1	4	50	19	8	4	-	92	83	23	42	66
Melton	-	-	-	8	-	2	2	1	-	-	9	1	2	1	-	3	1	2	1	-
North West Leics	-	-	1	35	1	1	-	-	-	1	23	18	2	-	-	26	71	3	14	2
Oadby & Wigston	-	-	1	65	-	7	5	5	-	2	23	8	1	-	-	22	34	2	6	3
Rutland	-	-	4	19	19	2	1	1	-	1	4	6	1	1	-	3	7	2	-	-

* Metropolitan county.
** Notification data are supplied in respect of local authority areas, and cannot be assigned individually to health areas (see note on page viii).
† Categories overlap and therefore some cases will be included in more than one column.
≠ See note on page vi.

Table 5 Series MB2 no.17

Table 5 - *continued*

Area	Typhoid fever	Paratyphoid fever	Dysentery (amoebic and bacillary)	Food poisoning		Tuberculosis (excluding chemoprophylaxis)					Whooping cough	Scarlet fever	Meningitis			Measles	Rubella	Viral hepatitis	Mumps	Malaria
				Formally notified	Ascertained by other means	All tuberculosis≠	All respiratory TB†	All pulmonary TB†	All TB meningitis†	Other forms of TB†			All meningitis	Meningococcal meningitis	Meningococcal septicaemia (without meningitis)					
Trent RHA - *continued*																				
Lincolnshire	-	-	2	566	170	16	13	13	-	3	154	103	16	8	2	141	130	22	56	5
Boston	-	-	-	143	-	2	2	2	-	-	19	17	1	-	-	14	8	2	7	-
East Lindsey	-	-	-	113	119	7	7	7	-	-	29	19	3	1	1	28	22	4	6	-
Lincoln	-	-	1	37	30	2	1	1	-	1	36	27	4	1	1	24	22	1	14	-
North Kesteven	-	-	1	64	-	1	1	1	-	-	27	2	2	2	-	14	16	3	7	-
South Holland	-	-	-	74	-	4	2	2	-	2	12	5	1	1	-	20	18	1	4	1
South Kesteven	-	-	-	96	-	-	-	-	-	-	24	6	1	-	-	31	36	9	10	3
West Lindsey	-	-	-	39	21	-	-	-	-	-	7	27	4	3	-	10	8	2	8	1
Nottinghamshire	1	1	68	678	466	89	68	68	1	22	209	145	55	28	6	169	225	170	90	12
Ashfield	1	-	-	50	-	6	4	4	-	2	11	55	8	3	-	15	71	5	7	-
Bassetlaw	-	-	-	57	42	8	8	8	-	-	36	12	5	4	3	18	24	4	17	-
Broxtowe	-	-	26	99	66	6	3	3	-	3	22	4	6	5	-	16	24	20	10	-
Gedling	-	-	8	170	19	2	2	2	-	-	15	21	7	3	-	14	30	30	11	1
Mansfield	-	-	10	28	8	10	7	7	-	3	24	7	8	1	-	16	17	27	7	1
Newark & Sherwood	-	-	1	73	19	3	3	3	-	-	28	8	5	3	-	22	15	13	7	1
Nottingham	-	1	23	160	234	47	37	37	-	11	18	25	12	7	3	56	26	66	18	8
Rushcliffe	-	-	-	41	78	7	4	4	1	3	55	13	4	2	-	12	18	5	13	1
East Anglian RHA																				
Cambridgeshire	1	2	25	316	60	50	45	45	1	4	185	57	16	6	1	153	160	73	83	11
Cambridge	1	2	14	91	1	7	7	7	-	-	8	7	-	-	-	9	-	11	4	4
East Cambridgeshire	-	-	1	30	8	-	-	-	-	-	3	2	1	-	-	8	9	3	23	-
Fenland	-	-	1	64	-	1	1	1	-	-	50	23	2	1	-	22	21	10	12	-
Huntingdonshire	-	-	-	43	37	12	11	11	-	1	64	7	7	1	-	33	39	7	19	1
Peterborough	-	-	3	35	-	27	23	23	1	3	26	4	4	2	-	55	81	23	20	4
South Cambridgeshire	-	-	6	53	14	3	3	3	-	-	34	14	2	2	1	26	10	19	5	2
Norfolk	-	1	15	375	68	26	17	15	-	9	238	49	30	12	4	103	115	26	64	5
Breckland	-	-	2	126	3	3	2	2	-	1	22	6	5	-	1	20	12	1	15	1
Broadland	-	-	-	33	-	3	1	1	-	2	27	12	3	1	-	9	12	-	6	-
Great Yarmouth	-	-	2	34	26	4	4	4	-	-	29	14	7	2	1	16	29	5	20	2
King's Lynn & West Norfolk	-	-	1	60	1	4	4	4	-	-	56	2	4	2	-	15	32	9	9	-
North Norfolk	-	-	-	23	-	4	1	1	-	3	7	7	2	2	-	20	-	2	2	-
Norwich	-	1	7	42	37	3	2	1	-	1	59	5	6	3	2	12	24	2	7	2
South Norfolk	-	-	3	57	1	5	3	2	-	2	38	3	3	2	-	11	6	7	5	-
Suffolk	-	-	7	473	126	21	11	11	2	9	85	80	30	16	1	107	105	34	50	6
Babergh	-	-	1	71	-	2	-	-	1	1	19	7	6	4	-	6	9	2	2	1
Forest Heath	-	-	-	29	-	-	-	-	-	-	6	3	3	2	-	8	7	7	6	-
Ipswich	-	-	2	116	27	3	2	2	-	1	30	14	6	4	-	26	20	9	15	1
Mid Suffolk	-	-	3	57	32	2	1	1	-	1	2	12	2	1	-	6	11	4	1	1
St Edmundsbury	-	-	1	40	16	-	-	-	-	-	11	8	4	1	-	6	27	6	10	1
Suffolk Coastal	-	-	-	46	-	6	6	6	-	1	9	26	2	-	-	8	16	3	9	1
Waveney	-	-	-	114	51	8	2	2	1	5	8	10	7	4	1	47	15	3	7	1
N W Thames RHA																				
Bedfordshire	6	2	35	426	225	53	34	31	2	18	116	61	17	6	-	144	67	52	34	18
Luton	5	2	22	200	108	29	18	15	-	12	40	21	11	2	-	64	32	17	18	15
Mid Bedfordshire	-	-	1	30	25	3	3	3	-	-	10	10	1	-	-	32	9	7	2	-
North Bedfordshire	1	-	8	17	30	12	9	9	-	3	16	4	1	1	-	28	14	14	10	3
South Bedfordshire	-	-	4	179	62	9	4	4	2	3	50	26	4	3	-	20	12	14	4	-
Hertfordshire	-	1	56	494	229	64	40	38	-	24	254	133	53	27	2	145	158	93	61	13
Broxbourne	-	-	4	12	30	4	2	2	-	2	19	7	2	2	-	13	15	10	5	-
Dacorum	-	-	-	19	33	9	5	5	-	4	10	4	6	4	-	14	12	9	6	-
East Hertfordshire	-	-	5	32	41	1	1	1	-	-	10	14	5	1	-	31	15	15	8	4
Hertsmere	-	-	14	114	13	5	3	3	-	2	56	37	9	5	1	15	9	6	9	1
North Hertfordshire	-	-	6	40	22	13	7	7	-	6	29	3	3	2	-	6	8	7	4	1
St Albans	-	-	3	58	4	5	3	1	-	2	25	25	5	4	1	17	6	6	3	3
Stevenage	-	-	4	21	21	5	4	4	-	1	29	10	6	-	-	5	9	3	1	-
Three Rivers	-	-	6	85	11	5	4	4	-	1	26	5	7	3	-	14	30	15	6	1
Watford	-	1	11	82	5	13	9	9	-	4	22	1	5	3	-	23	26	10	10	3
Welwyn Hatfield	-	-	3	31	49	4	2	2	-	2	28	27	5	3	-	7	28	12	9	-

†   Categories overlap and therefore some cases will be included in more than one column.
≠   See note on page vi.

Table 5 - *continued*

Area	Typhoid fever	Paratyphoid fever	Dysentery (amoebic and bacillary)	Food poisoning Formally notified	Food poisoning Ascertained by other means	Tuberculosis All tuberculosis≠	All respiratory TB†	All pulmonary TB†	All TB meningitis†	Other forms of TB†	Whooping cough	Scarlet fever	Meningitis All meningitis	Meningococcal meningitis	Meningococcal septicaemia (without meningitis)	Measles	Rubella	Viral hepatitis	Mumps	Malaria
NW Thames RHA - *continued*																				
Surrey (pt)	-	-	8	42	1	5	3	3	-	3	7	1	2	1	-	6	3	-	3	2
Spelthorne	-	-	8	42	1	5	3	3	-	3	7	1	2	1	-	6	3	-	3	2
Greater London (pt)	34	10	198	1,545	276	523	388	358	1	139	348	198	67	33	15	326	216	158	92	305
Barnet	1	1	37	436	76	73	49	49	-	24	64	37	15	4	1	49	50	32	21	38
Brent	6	1	27	100	53	95	67	64	-	28	27	5	4	2	2	29	12	23	11	90
Ealing	15	2	40	95	35	87	60	58	-	28	53	62	6	4	5	40	36	23	7	34
Hammersmith & Fulham	2	1	11	66	32	41	41	41	-	-	24	10	9	4	2	7	11	13	2	20
Harrow	-	1	15	341	13	66	47	29	1	21	39	42	9	6	1	27	19	17	15	14
Hillingdon	2	1	13	162	14	32	24	22	-	8	87	17	4	1	-	109	50	8	22	34
Hounslow	3	-	5	97	-	37	23	19	-	14	38	15	7	2	3	47	29	8	9	19
Kensington & Chelsea	2	2	19	79	12	38	30	30	-	9	10	5	4	3	-	5	1	22	4	18
Westminster, City of**	3	1	31	169	41	54	47	46	-	7	6	5	9	7	1	13	8	12	1	38
N E Thames RHA																				
Essex	-	1	60	1,519	288	47	34	32	3	10	479	323	58	24	6	471	315	167	93	7
Basildon	-	-	5	234	-	5	5	5	-	-	45	16	7	5	4	25	12	5	7	-
Braintree	-	-	3	124	87	5	4	4	-	1	41	26	2	1	-	42	40	5	6	-
Brentwood	-	-	3	70	27	2	1	1	-	1	22	41	3	3	-	5	7	8	9	-
Castle Point	-	-	-	18	-	-	-	-	-	-	8	2	1	-	-	73	17	-	11	-
Chelmsford	-	-	17	116	115	4	1	1	2	1	89	45	5	3	1	18	49	11	15	-
Colchester	-	-	-	210	-	2	2	2	-	-	51	10	3	1	-	16	27	15	5	-
Epping Forest	-	-	-	40	-	5	3	3	-	2	28	9	8	1	1	22	29	12	7	2
Harlow	-	1	-	34	-	5	4	4	1	-	42	20	4	-	-	21	18	4	5	3
Maldon	-	-	-	26	16	-	-	-	-	-	6	7	-	-	-	23	13	6	1	-
Rochford	-	-	1	19	38	2	1	1	-	1	3	11	4	-	-	24	4	9	3	-
Southend-on-Sea	-	-	-	126	-	8	8	7	-	-	29	6	3	1	-	76	49	6	16	-
Tendring	-	-	-	118	-	1	-	-	-	1	15	22	8	5	-	20	10	7	2	-
Thurrock	-	-	21	303	5	7	4	4	-	3	74	91	7	3	-	94	33	59	3	2
Uttlesford	-	-	10	81	-	1	1	-	-	-	26	17	3	1	-	12	7	20	3	-
Greater London (pt)	25	11	149	1,237	487	623	496	417	7	125	441	219	110	42	11	493	252	260	155	225
City of London	-	-	-	1	2	-	-	-	-	-	-	-	-	-	-	-	-	1	-	-
Barking & Dagenham	-	3	6	45	48	18	14	14	-	4	39	10	8	3	1	70	5	4	13	4
Camden	6	1	28	163	-	64	57	55	1	6	21	10	9	5	1	15	6	16	3	40
Enfield	2	-	11	190	150	25	15	15	-	10	76	54	9	3	-	39	55	22	24	16
Hackney	2	-	10	117	-	78	76	51	-	2	39	6	10	5	-	14	20	45	12	41
Haringey	3	-	16	162	-	65	63	51	1	1	44	12	8	3	2	57	12	29	21	34
Havering	-	-	9	64	69	8	7	2	-	1	35	34	6	3	-	73	33	8	21	1
Islington	-	1	18	170	27	44	31	30	-	16	27	24	13	6	2	13	24	28	12	13
Newham	4	-	16	107	-	133	82	78	2	50	67	13	16	4	3	61	38	25	26	38
Redbridge	4	1	2	49	21	41	32	25	1	8	15	25	8	3	1	19	15	12	5	11
Tower Hamlets	2	5	16	161	-	94	83	67	1	11	35	9	13	2	1	79	20	52	11	15
Waltham Forest	2	-	16	7	170	53	36	29	1	16	43	22	10	5	-	53	24	18	7	12
S E Thames RHA																				
East Sussex	1	-	25	518	278	40	37	37	-	3	148	66	19	5	-	84	92	62	49	6
Brighton	1	-	6	96	38	17	17	17	-	-	28	24	1	-	-	23	9	12	4	4
Eastbourne	-	-	1	23	-	3	1	1	-	2	18	10	4	-	-	5	10	4	4	-
Hastings	-	-	-	56	3	4	4	4	-	-	37	1	2	1	-	20	16	13	9	1
Hove	-	-	4	108	63	5	5	5	-	-	33	18	4	2	-	14	-	13	3	-
Lewes	-	-	-	94	68	4	3	3	-	1	14	-	1	-	-	7	26	8	19	1
Rother	-	-	5	75	-	2	2	2	-	-	5	3	4	2	-	10	14	3	1	-
Wealden	-	-	9	66	106	5	5	5	-	-	13	10	3	-	-	5	17	9	9	-
Kent	4	-	55	1,059	404	80	55	49	5	21	559	294	83	33	4	556	482	654	134	33
Ashford	2	-	5	168	3	5	1	-	2	2	53	15	4	2	-	49	35	23	24	2
Canterbury	-	-	6	55	29	7	6	4	-	1	44	8	5	4	-	28	12	12	3	-
Dartford	-	-	4	54	104	5	3	3	-	2	44	35	3	-	-	45	46	16	15	4
Dover	-	-	1	63	70	5	2	2	-	3	38	8	6	2	-	45	37	17	5	3
Gillingham	-	-	3	10	-	5	5	5	-	-	16	6	1	1	-	23	39	8	5	5

** Notification data are supplied in respect of local authority areas, and cannot be assigned individually to health areas (see note on page viii).
Categories overlap and therefore some cases will be included in more than one column.
≠ See note on page vi.

Table 5 Series MB2 no.17

Table 5 - *continued*

Area	Typhoid fever	Paratyphoid fever	Dysentery (amoebic and bacillary)	Food poisoning		Tuberculosis (excluding chemoprophylaxis)					Whooping cough	Scarlet fever	Meningitis			Measles	Rubella	Viral hepatitis	Mumps	Malaria
				Formally notified	Ascertained by other means	All tuberculosis≠	All respiratory TB†	All pulmonary TB†	All TB meningitis†	Other forms of TB†			All meningitis	Meningococcal meningitis	Meningococcal septicaemia (without meningitis)					
SE Thames RHA - *continued*																				
Gravesham	1	-	2	19	125	6	5	5	-	1	27	11	7	2	1	29	32	13	6	5
Maidstone	-	-	10	82	-	5	2	2	1	2	49	62	10	5	2	30	17	63	3	-
Rochester upon Medway	-	-	2	117	-	3	2	2	-	1	51	4	15	8	-	99	65	50	15	8
Sevenoaks	-	-	-	71	20	4	3	2	-	2	36	18	5	-	-	33	37	47	9	2
Shepway	-	-	-	120	15	9	9	7	-	-	37	9	2	1	-	40	40	267	6	1
Swale	-	-	6	97	-	9	5	5	2	2	68	58	7	3	1	62	29	51	15	1
Thanet	-	-	5	75	16	9	7	7	-	2	52	14	3	2	-	39	54	8	14	2
Tonbridge & Malling	1	-	8	60	-	4	3	3	-	1	18	16	8	2	-	19	26	28	10	-
Tunbridge Wells	-	-	3	68	22	4	2	2	-	2	26	30	7	1	-	15	13	51	4	-
Greater London (pt)	5	2	51	925	98	262	204	194	1	57	262	165	66	33	5	314	247	221	101	88
Bexley	1	-	5	237	-	18	12	10	1	5	62	49	20	9	2	48	63	44	32	4
Bromley	-	2	3	103	97	16	11	11	-	5	88	65	10	5	-	70	73	47	24	12
Greenwich	1	-	13	224	-	30	22	22	-	8	26	8	12	10	-	37	60	79	20	4
Lambeth	2	-	12	203	-	77	58	57	-	19	30	3	5	-	1	84	19	25	18	29
Lewisham	-	-	-	59	1	46	46	42	-	-	24	32	9	5	-	33	18	10	5	12
Southwark	1	-	18	99	-	75	55	52	-	20	32	8	10	4	2	42	14	16	2	27
S W Thames RHA																				
Hampshire (pt)	1	-	6	235	-	3	3	3	-	-	55	23	7	4	-	20	30	15	13	4
Hart**	1	-	5	132	-	1	1	1	-	-	20	9	3	3	-	5	22	12	8	2
Rushmoor	-	-	1	103	-	2	2	2	-	-	35	14	4	1	-	15	8	3	5	2
Surrey (pt)	3	3	56	768	361	36	30	28	-	6	139	61	26	11	4	95	74	63	38	21
Elmbridge	-	-	2	167	63	6	5	5	-	1	18	3	4	1	-	10	-	5	4	5
Epsom & Ewell	-	-	2	50	8	7	6	6	-	1	15	7	5	3	-	17	6	4	4	4
Guildford	1	-	3	57	50	5	4	4	-	1	24	-	7	4	1	11	22	13	2	5
Mole Valley	-	2	8	135	103	1	-	-	-	1	2	10	-	-	-	9	15	9	3	2
Reigate & Banstead	-	-	12	96	-	6	5	4	-	1	17	8	2	1	3	20	2	14	6	2
Runnymede	-	-	-	45	-	3	3	3	-	-	5	3	1	1	-	7	4	1	6	-
Surrey Heath	-	-	-	51	-	-	-	-	-	-	13	2	3	1	-	4	7	5	1	1
Tandridge	-	-	8	58	38	4	4	3	-	-	17	17	3	-	-	8	7	2	4	2
Waverley	-	1	9	80	78	1	1	1	-	-	11	6	-	-	-	2	7	6	3	-
Woking	2	-	12	29	21	3	2	2	-	1	17	5	1	-	-	7	4	4	5	-
West Sussex	1	-	31	395	447	24	17	17	3	7	218	83	23	6	3	84	40	36	31	13
Adur	-	-	1	22	7	1	1	1	-	-	21	12	2	-	-	7	4	-	4	-
Arun	-	-	7	62	54	8	5	5	3	3	38	7	3	-	-	15	4	2	2	-
Chichester	-	-	5	12	46	1	-	-	-	1	12	4	4	1	1	13	5	4	1	-
Crawley	-	-	12	72	104	5	3	3	-	2	66	5	6	2	1	20	8	6	7	11
Horsham	-	-	3	98	71	6	5	5	-	1	17	19	4	1	-	7	9	10	6	1
Mid Sussex	-	-	3	83	147	1	1	1	-	-	34	33	2	1	-	14	9	8	10	1
Worthing	1	-	-	46	18	2	2	2	-	-	30	3	2	1	1	8	1	6	1	-
Greater London (pt)	7	1	84	762	105	195	137	134	1	57	181	183	49	25	5	238	221	128	61	75
Croydon	2	-	8	111	-	60	41	41	-	19	37	34	16	6	-	69	42	31	12	20
Kingston upon Thames	-	-	3	50	-	13	7	7	-	6	13	8	3	-	-	23	8	4	6	4
Merton	-	1	16	189	47	27	19	19	-	8	18	66	6	4	-	33	15	16	11	13
Richmond upon Thames	1	-	12	53	17	8	7	6	-	1	21	21	5	3	1	10	16	7	5	5
Sutton	2	-	12	212	22	17	13	13	-	4	67	42	9	8	3	53	117	28	14	2
Wandsworth	2	-	33	147	19	70	50	48	1	19	25	12	10	4	1	50	23	42	13	31
Wessex RHA																				
Avon (pt)	-	-	1	57	-	9	7	7	-	2	55	23	6	3	-	20	15	7	8	1
Bath	-	-	1	34	-	6	5	5	-	1	37	16	1	-	-	7	8	2	1	-
Wansdyke**	-	-	-	23	-	3	2	2	-	1	18	7	5	3	-	13	7	5	7	1
Dorset	-	1	21	156	567	26	22	22	-	4	139	108	18	8	1	136	76	68	54	4
Bournemouth	-	-	6	33	171	8	5	5	-	3	45	23	7	2	-	25	23	22	16	1
Christchurch	-	-	2	4	39	1	1	1	-	-	3	3	1	1	1	2	-	1	4	-
East Dorset	-	1	1	8	60	5	5	5	-	-	6	2	2	1	-	-	5	9	4	-
North Dorset	-	-	-	24	8	3	3	3	-	-	6	21	1	-	-	13	7	5	3	1
Poole	-	-	6	25	220	4	4	4	-	-	35	10	4	2	-	23	27	23	12	1
Purbeck	-	-	3	17	41	-	-	-	-	-	14	7	1	1	-	66	4	2	6	-
West Dorset	-	-	2	12	22	4	3	3	-	1	21	34	-	-	-	6	8	2	4	-
Weymouth & Portland	-	-	1	33	6	1	1	1	-	-	9	8	2	1	-	1	2	4	5	1

** Notification data are supplied in respect of local authority areas, and cannot be assigned individually to health areas (see note on page viii).
† Categories overlap and therefore some cases will be included in more than one column.
≠ See note on page vi.

Table 5 - *continued*

Area	Typhoid fever	Paratyphoid fever	Dysentery (amoebic and bacillary)	Food poisoning		Tuberculosis (excluding chemoprophylaxis)					Whooping cough	Scarlet fever	Meningitis			Measles	Rubella	Viral hepatitis	Mumps	Malaria
				Formally notified	Ascertained by other means	All tuberculosis≠	All respiratory TB†	All pulmonary TB†	All TB meningitis†	Other forms of TB†			All meningitis	Meningococcal meningitis	Meningococcal septicaemia (without meningitis)					
Wessex RHA - *continued*																				
Hampshire (pt)	-	-	21	787	446	47	31	25	-	16	312	138	57	31	4	196	184	63	128	16
Basingstoke & Deane	-	-	4	124	1	-	-	-	-	-	50	11	8	4	-	14	9	10	10	-
East Hampshire	-	-	-	102	-	2	2	2	-	-	34	15	2	1	1	17	23	3	10	-
Eastleigh	-	-	-	38	25	6	6	6	-	-	12	15	3	2	-	11	2	2	3	1
Fareham	-	-	-	63	-	1	1	1	-	-	24	10	6	4	1	33	39	7	13	2
Gosport	-	-	-	39	57	3	3	3	-	-	6	-	6	2	-	9	7	8	9	2
Havant	-	-	-	47	-	2	1	1	-	1	51	13	4	2	-	24	26	4	24	2
New Forest	-	-	1	79	69	3	2	2	-	1	30	17	5	3	1	28	26	3	12	-
Portsmouth	-	-	3	111	2	6	-	-	-	6	38	11	10	7	1	19	18	5	10	2
Southampton	-	-	8	77	138	21	13	7	-	8	39	29	10	5	-	25	14	15	25	5
Test Valley	-	-	2	74	-	2	2	2	-	-	19	14	1	-	-	12	18	5	5	1
Winchester	-	-	3	33	154	1	1	1	-	-	9	3	2	1	-	4	2	1	7	1
Isle of Wight	-	-	4	9	131	5	5	5	-	-	45	14	6	3	2	31	31	2	15	-
Medina	-	-	2	8	91	3	3	3	-	-	24	7	5	2	2	18	18	-	10	-
South Wight	-	-	2	1	40	2	2	2	-	-	21	7	1	1	-	13	13	2	5	-
Wiltshire	-	-	38	559	3	24	19	19	1	5	125	68	20	4	-	90	105	34	70	12
Kennet	-	-	1	62	-	2	2	2	-	-	7	3	-	-	-	8	13	5	4	4
North Wiltshire	-	-	4	90	-	1	1	1	-	-	27	12	1	-	-	20	18	1	20	-
Salisbury	-	-	3	128	3	6	5	5	-	1	6	12	2	-	-	15	15	13	16	1
Thamesdown	-	-	29	268	-	12	9	9	1	3	54	23	17	4	-	28	47	14	26	7
West Wiltshire	-	-	1	11	-	3	2	2	-	1	31	18	-	-	-	19	12	1	4	-
Oxford RHA																				
Berkshire	4	2	69	870	88	72	48	48	14	11	155	102	43	20	9	142	185	329	58	21
Bracknell Forest	-	-	5	199	5	5	4	4	-	1	32	44	10	3	-	26	91	16	15	-
Newbury	-	-	6	98	26	1	1	1	-	-	45	11	7	3	2	16	35	63	9	-
Reading	1	-	6	32	20	20	14	14	-	6	21	1	10	6	3	7	9	116	5	4
Slough	3	1	21	170	4	35	24	24	8	3	27	12	6	3	1	45	10	31	15	13
Windsor & Maidenhead	-	-	6	273	8	10	4	4	6	1	12	24	2	1	1	26	14	42	3	3
Wokingham	-	1	25	98	25	1	1	1	-	-	18	10	8	4	2	22	26	61	11	1
Buckinghamshire	2	-	47	552	4	19	7	7	-	13	159	61	10	3	3	68	135	67	53	13
Aylesbury Vale	-	-	3	68	-	4	3	3	-	1	40	22	-	-	1	26	32	15	19	3
Chiltern	-	-	13	94	-	3	1	1	-	2	16	3	-	-	-	5	6	24	2	2
Milton Keynes	-	-	9	252	1	3	-	-	-	3	69	28	3	1	-	26	73	6	25	6
South Bucks	-	-	6	37	3	3	1	1	-	2	18	1	1	1	-	8	15	8	6	2
Wycombe	2	-	16	101	-	6	2	2	-	5	16	7	6	1	2	3	9	14	1	-
Northamptonshire	2	-	15	592	104	52	42	39	1	9	134	62	31	9	4	113	66	247	40	12
Corby	-	-	5	64	33	4	4	2	-	-	8	3	6	3	1	28	15	217	2	3
Daventry	-	-	-	41	3	-	-	-	-	-	12	4	3	1	-	4	3	-	2	-
East Northants	-	-	1	16	-	4	4	4	-	-	30	2	4	1	1	8	10	5	4	-
Kettering	-	-	1	97	-	4	2	1	-	2	19	18	4	1	-	27	22	8	12	2
Northampton	1	-	8	312	25	26	21	21	-	5	25	27	8	1	2	27	7	9	10	4
South Northants	1	-	-	42	1	-	-	-	-	-	9	4	1	-	-	10	4	3	1	1
Wellingborough	-	-	-	20	42	14	11	11	1	2	31	4	5	2	-	9	5	5	9	2
Oxfordshire	-	2	40	177	292	21	20	20	-	1	105	73	31	10	4	62	55	69	42	12
Cherwell	-	-	4	28	48	4	3	3	-	1	11	3	9	4	-	10	17	9	8	2
Oxford	-	2	18	47	74	5	5	5	-	-	11	16	4	1	1	18	3	15	6	5
South Oxfordshire	-	-	4	27	63	5	5	5	-	-	31	8	10	2	2	15	8	35	9	1
Vale of White Horse	-	-	6	37	54	4	4	4	-	-	34	43	4	2	-	6	15	4	12	3
West Oxfordshire	-	-	8	38	53	3	3	3	-	-	18	3	4	1	1	13	12	6	7	1
South Western RHA																				
Avon (pt)	2	2	142	630	449	35	33	31	1	1	197	125	76	27	11	125	259	50	77	20
Bristol	2	1	126	239	336	31	29	27	1	1	74	70	53	13	4	68	153	41	36	14
Kingswood	-	-	1	73	2	1	1	1	-	-	29	3	5	-	1	14	19	3	9	-
Northavon	-	1	3	50	70	3	3	3	-	-	59	11	9	9	1	21	63	4	20	3
Woodspring	-	-	12	268	41	-	-	-	-	-	35	41	9	5	5	22	24	2	12	3
Cornwall & Isles of Scilly	-	-	9	272	232	10	6	6	-	4	253	58	16	7	3	111	222	114	41	8
Caradon	-	-	1	68	17	2	2	2	-	-	32	9	2	2	1	24	61	12	7	1
Carrick	-	-	7	52	101	4	2	2	-	2	54	14	7	1	-	9	10	2	5	5
Kerrier	-	-	1	39	12	1	1	1	-	-	102	18	2	1	-	27	38	78	13	1

†   Categories overlap and therefore some cases will be included in more than one column.

≠   See note on page vi

Table 5 Series MB2 no.17

Table 5 - *continued*

Area	Typhoid fever	Paratyphoid fever	Dysentery (amoebic and bacillary)	Food poisoning Formally notified	Food poisoning Ascertained by other means	All tuberculosis≠	All respiratory TB†	All pulmonary TB†	All TB meningitis†	Other forms of TB†	Whooping cough	Scarlet fever	All meningitis	Meningococcal meningitis	Meningococcal septicaemia (without meningitis)	Measles	Rubella	Viral hepatitis	Mumps	Malaria
South Western RHA - *continued*																				
North Cornwall	-	-	-	21	52	-	-	-	-	-	26	10	2	2	2	13	46	5	4	1
Penwith	-	-	-	50	50	1	-	-	-	1	13	4	2	-	-	14	31	13	7	-
Restormel	-	-	-	42	-	2	1	1	-	1	26	3	1	1	-	24	36	4	5	-
Isles of Scilly	-	-	-	-	-	-	-	-	-	-	-	-	-	-	-	-	-	-	-	-
Devon	-	-	23	1,099	490	33	27	24	1	5	232	79	59	30	5	160	143	89	73	2
East Devon	-	-	-	20	4	-	-	-	-	-	3	10	4	1	1	8	7	7	3	1
Exeter	-	-	-	38	29	9	9	9	-	-	38	16	9	6	-	33	19	6	10	1
Mid Devon	-	-	2	15	2	1	1	1	-	-	14	5	6	1	-	11	7	10	9	-
North Devon	-	-	2	196	-	3	3	3	-	-	22	3	1	1	-	9	5	9	5	-
Plymouth	-	-	6	361	128	9	7	4	-	2	76	21	19	13	2	54	71	15	31	-
South Hams	-	-	3	151	74	-	-	-	-	-	22	12	5	3	-	8	11	11	-	-
Teignbridge	-	-	2	70	90	6	3	3	1	2	20	1	5	2	-	13	2	13	2	-
Torbay	-	-	5	144	156	4	3	3	-	1	30	11	5	1	2	11	16	12	10	-
Torridge	-	-	2	23	7	1	1	1	-	-	4	-	3	1	-	7	-	3	1	-
West Devon	-	-	1	81	-	-	-	-	-	-	3	-	2	1	-	6	5	3	2	-
Gloucestershire	-	-	8	337	101	23	17	12	-	6	195	80	35	19	2	113	78	124	55	5
Cheltenham	-	-	-	51	-	-	-	-	-	-	24	13	10	3	-	14	4	1	2	2
Cotswold	-	-	2	75	-	1	1	1	-	-	16	8	1	-	-	14	14	1	6	1
Forest of Dean	-	-	1	28	-	2	1	1	-	1	60	6	4	3	-	26	15	6	22	1
Gloucester	-	-	4	80	54	11	8	7	-	3	37	7	6	3	1	31	15	105	10	1
Stroud	-	-	1	45	47	5	4	2	-	1	40	29	4	2	1	13	8	5	6	-
Tewkesbury	-	-	-	58	-	4	3	1	-	1	18	17	10	8	-	15	22	6	9	-
Somerset	-	1	6	172	-	13	9	8	-	4	85	54	2	2	-	131	146	22	64	4
Mendip**	-	-	3	49	-	1	1	1	-	-	22	20	2	2	-	21	21	10	16	1
Sedgemoor	-	-	2	45	-	3	3	3	-	-	26	9	-	-	-	40	38	4	14	2
South Somerset	-	-	-	50	-	4	3	3	-	1	17	17	-	-	-	41	32	2	13	-
Taunton Deane	-	1	1	25	-	5	2	1	-	3	14	8	-	-	-	19	31	6	16	1
West Somerset	-	-	-	3	-	-	-	-	-	-	6	-	-	-	-	10	24	-	5	-
West Midlands RHA																				
West Midlands*	19	15	158	1,342	1,826	561	398	380	6	169	757	425	178	79	15	959	607	416	277	119
Birmingham	9	7	84	307	401	289	197	196	1	100	314	161	76	29	10	187	196	152	103	48
Coventry	2	3	28	253	380	54	40	32	3	11	83	18	23	19	3	185	93	79	33	31
Dudley	2	-	4	168	726	35	30	27	-	6	106	33	18	9	-	85	80	51	33	5
Sandwell	4	2	32	14	180	61	37	36	-	24	81	49	17	7	-	154	80	39	32	9
Solihull	-	-	3	26	138	6	5	5	-	1	39	58	11	3	-	57	41	27	13	-
Walsall	1	2	5	238	1	49	41	36	-	8	70	79	17	3	2	189	61	59	24	9
Wolverhampton	1	1	2	336	-	67	48	48	2	19	64	27	16	9	-	102	56	9	39	17
Hereford & Worcester	2	-	21	506	110	31	18	18	-	13	149	133	28	16	-	142	148	36	90	8
Bromsgrove	-	-	4	41	-	1	1	1	-	-	30	6	4	2	-	14	15	4	4	2
Hereford	-	-	-	23	-	1	1	1	-	-	3	2	-	-	-	7	14	-	2	2
Leominster	-	-	-	29	-	-	-	-	-	-	14	-	-	-	-	7	9	2	3	-
Malvern Hills	-	-	2	174	-	7	3	3	-	4	9	10	5	4	-	17	3	8	5	1
Redditch	2	-	2	39	3	1	1	1	-	-	26	14	5	1	-	21	40	2	6	1
South Herefordshire	-	-	3	46	-	2	1	1	-	1	6	9	2	2	-	4	24	4	58	1
Worcester	-	-	5	59	47	9	7	7	-	2	7	14	5	4	-	18	3	4	2	1
Wychavon	-	-	4	57	50	7	2	2	-	5	16	7	2	-	-	18	8	5	5	-
Wyre Forest	-	-	1	38	10	3	2	2	-	1	38	71	5	3	-	36	32	7	5	-
Shropshire	-	1	6	204	76	27	19	18	3	6	241	76	22	10	7	91	90	19	63	5
Bridgnorth	-	-	-	18	8	2	2	2	-	-	10	35	-	-	-	3	5	-	7	-
North Shropshire	-	-	-	24	14	3	3	3	-	-	16	3	2	1	2	11	22	2	6	-
Oswestry	-	-	-	5	5	-	-	-	-	-	21	-	-	-	-	5	8	1	15	-
Shrewsbury & Atcham	-	-	3	36	20	-	-	-	-	-	35	17	8	2	2	17	8	3	17	-
South Shropshire	-	-	-	34	1	3	1	1	2	-	25	2	1	1	-	7	4	7	-	-
The Wrekin	-	1	3	87	28	19	13	12	1	6	134	19	11	6	3	48	43	6	18	5
Staffordshire	2	-	8	302	437	73	44	41	1	28	178	101	12	2	1	332	246	37	99	6
Cannock Chase	-	-	-	14	-	5	3	3	1	1	8	25	2	1	-	43	14	-	15	-
East Staffordshire	-	-	2	55	1	9	3	3	-	6	17	9	2	1	-	12	17	21	2	5
Lichfield	-	-	5	72	51	-	-	-	-	-	15	17	2	-	-	56	52	10	16	-
Newcastle-under-Lyme	-	-	-	38	43	8	6	6	-	2	30	4	2	-	-	33	9	1	5	-
South Staffordshire	-	-	1	58	-	3	3	3	-	-	32	4	1	-	-	23	33	2	9	1

*   Metropolitan county.
** Notification data are supplied in respect of local authority areas, and cannot be assigned individually to health areas (see note on page viii).
†   Categories overlap and therefore some cases will be included in more than one column.
≠   See note on page vi.

Area	Typhoid fever	Paratyphoid fever	Dysentery (amoebic and bacillary)	Food poisoning		Tuberculosis (excluding chemoprophylaxis)					Whooping cough	Scarlet fever	Meningitis			Measles	Rubella	Viral hepatitis	Mumps	Malaria
				Formally notified	Ascertained by other means	All tuberculosis≠	All respiratory TB†	All pulmonary TB†	All TB meningitis†	Other forms of TB†			All meningitis	Meningococcal meningitis	Meningococcal septicaemia (without meningitis)					
West Midlands RHA - continued																				
Stafford	-	-	-	-	250	6	5	5	-	1	18	8	1	-	1	21	46	1	13	-
Staffordshire Moorlands	-	-	-	37	-	8	4	1	-	4	15	27	-	-	-	14	5	-	15	-
Stoke-on-Trent	2	-	-	20	56	34	20	20	-	14	35	4	2	-	-	69	53	1	16	-
Tamworth	-	-	-	8	36	-	-	-	-	-	8	3	-	-	-	61	17	1	8	-
Warwickshire	-	-	5	477	99	40	32	31	-	8	132	89	22	9	-	154	119	62	39	10
North Warwickshire	-	-	-	84	-	6	4	4	-	2	11	15	5	1	-	13	26	2	5	-
Nuneaton & Bedworth	-	-	-	165	-	10	10	9	-	-	57	8	13	5	-	85	27	40	16	4
Rugby	-	-	2	53	4	9	7	7	-	2	28	24	3	3	-	33	28	3	9	-
Stratford-on-Avon	-	-	1	96	45	7	5	5	-	2	16	12	1	-	-	14	17	5	6	2
Warwick	-	-	2	79	50	8	6	6	-	2	20	30	-	-	-	9	21	12	3	4
Mersey RHA																				
Merseyside*	-	-	26	1,101	70	97	81	81	-	17	560	222	118	58	19	426	212	455	112	9
Knowsley	-	-	-	51	11	8	5	5	-	3	78	42	17	12	3	52	26	26	11	-
Liverpool	-	-	22	260	58	54	48	48	-	7	167	67	32	17	10	162	62	343	30	8
St Helens	-	-	3	135	-	9	5	5	-	4	60	41	18	6	-	49	32	15	17	-
Sefton	-	-	-	100	1	12	12	12	-	-	68	19	10	6	1	56	15	37	16	-
Wirral	-	-	1	555	-	14	11	11	-	3	187	53	41	17	5	107	77	34	38	1
Cheshire	1	2	9	569	73	42	32	29	-	10	388	156	44	20	9	240	267	48	80	6
Chester	-	-	-	49	47	3	3	3	-	-	25	11	2	2	1	13	21	5	6	-
Congleton	-	-	4	55	-	1	1	1	-	-	50	11	-	-	2	18	12	2	1	1
Crewe and Nantwich	1	1	-	88	3	4	3	3	-	1	44	2	3	1	-	22	23	1	10	-
Ellesmere Port & Neston	-	-	-	39	23	2	2	2	-	-	52	21	2	1	-	17	11	5	9	-
Halton	-	-	2	64	-	7	2	2	-	5	46	24	18	6	4	76	99	12	17	1
Macclesfield	-	-	1	68	-	5	2	2	-	3	52	8	8	5	-	23	25	13	8	3
Vale Royal	-	-	2	78	-	-	-	-	-	-	54	31	4	3	-	6	18	3	3	-
Warrington	-	1	-	128	-	20	19	16	-	1	65	48	7	2	2	65	58	7	26	1
North Western RHA																				
Greater Manchester*	7	9	190	1,044	1,146	405	328	317	7	71	1,083	240	182	87	21	912	783	702	256	56
Bolton	-	-	40	121	549	90	86	86	-	4	85	44	23	8	9	64	63	84	19	8
Bury	-	-	8	152	-	23	18	18	-	5	107	5	4	3	-	45	21	149	5	10
Manchester	3	3	50	169	2	87	71	70	-	16	137	36	36	21	1	94	127	80	41	16
Oldham	-	1	10	24	-	42	31	30	3	9	113	12	9	7	2	67	32	24	14	5
Rochdale	1	1	8	86	19	40	26	26	2	12	64	32	8	3	3	43	57	126	13	5
Salford	-	1	28	225	38	28	24	24	-	4	86	5	12	7	2	69	76	21	14	2
Stockport	1	1	6	97	217	22	18	17	-	4	113	16	15	12	-	61	31	43	18	-
Tameside	1	-	11	20	62	26	26	18	-	-	93	25	25	9	2	211	70	73	43	4
Trafford	1	2	29	52	255	29	15	15	-	14	76	16	8	3	1	55	127	43	36	4
Wigan	-	-	-	98	4	18	13	13	2	3	209	49	42	14	1	203	179	59	53	2
Lancashire	8	3	81	1,092	493	199	126	115	2	72	370	166	75	46	8	468	367	342	148	23
Blackburn	4	1	15	57	-	42	10	9	-	32	34	5	4	2	-	84	48	60	3	3
Blackpool	-	-	6	117	179	9	8	8	-	1	22	7	9	5	1	43	22	4	5	1
Burnley	-	1	30	191	-	17	11	9	-	6	24	1	5	3	1	22	30	85	7	1
Chorley	1	-	-	54	136	6	6	5	-	-	38	40	4	3	2	42	65	2	88	1
Fylde	-	-	-	69	128	1	1	-	-	-	6	7	5	3	-	13	7	3	3	-
Hyndburn	-	-	8	47	-	9	6	6	-	3	4	4	2	1	1	29	24	38	2	2
Lancaster	-	-	1	28	5	10	10	9	-	-	15	11	9	6	-	3	1	34	2	-
Pendle	1	-	17	135	-	35	33	33	1	1	18	9	6	3	-	32	6	37	-	10
Preston	2	1	4	42	36	51	31	28	1	20	36	31	2	-	-	52	46	22	11	4
Ribble Valley	-	-	-	79	1	4	3	2	-	1	24	5	2	1	-	5	18	2	1	-
Rossendale	-	-	-	133	-	7	2	2	-	5	37	10	2	1	-	35	23	29	8	-
South Ribble	-	-	-	32	-	5	3	3	-	2	17	32	8	3	1	18	23	3	2	-
West Lancashire	-	-	-	42	-	1	-	-	-	1	91	2	11	9	1	66	32	17	14	-
Wyre	-	-	-	66	8	2	2	1	-	-	4	2	6	6	1	24	22	6	2	1

* Metropolitan county.
≠ Categories overlap and therefore some cases will be included in more than one column.
† See note on page vi.

Table 5 Series MB2 no.17

Table 5 - *continued*

Area	Typhoid fever	Paratyphoid fever	Dysentery (amoebic and bacillary)	Food poisoning Formally notified	Food poisoning Ascertained by other means	All tuberculosis≠	All respiratory TB†	All pulmonary TB†	All TB meningitis†	Other forms of TB†	Whooping cough	Scarlet fever	All meningitis	Meningococcal meningitis	Meningococcal septicaemia (without meningitis)	Measles	Rubella	Viral hepatitis	Mumps	Malaria
Wales																				
Clwyd	-	-	10	710	2	28	27	21	-	1	98	23	35	14	-	52	34	18	15	2
Alyn and Deeside	-	-	-	84	-	3	3	3	-	-	41	4	3	2	-	6	14	1	3	1
Colwyn	-	-	-	90	-	1	1	1	-	-	10	4	3	1	-	15	2	1	1	-
Delyn	-	-	1	127	-	3	3	3	-	-	9	2	5	2	-	1	3	2	3	-
Glyndwr	-	-	-	94	-	4	4	3	-	-	9	1	3	-	-	-	6	3	-	1
Rhuddlan	-	-	1	65	-	5	5	5	-	-	11	12	6	1	-	3	2	7	1	-
Wrexham Maelor	-	-	8	250	2	12	11	6	-	1	18	-	15	8	-	27	7	4	7	-
Dyfed	-	-	5	136	145	32	27	27	1	4	139	31	48	14	3	52	37	10	30	2
Carmarthen	-	-	1	42	10	1	1	1	-	-	13	1	9	3	-	8	9	-	14	1
Ceredigion	-	-	2	29	40	5	5	5	-	-	26	5	-	-	-	4	-	2	4	-
Dinefwr	-	-	-	11	10	4	4	4	-	-	34	1	1	-	-	8	10	1	-	-
Llanelli	-	-	-	18	7	6	6	6	-	-	45	3	5	3	1	11	9	2	4	-
Preseli Pembrokeshire	-	-	1	29	17	13	8	8	1	4	10	16	6	5	2	20	8	1	7	1
South Pembrokeshire	-	-	1	7	61	3	3	3	-	-	11	5	27	3	-	1	1	4	1	-
Gwent	1	-	-	96	1	20	16	15	1	3	195	37	34	15	10	120	68	33	62	1
Blaenau Gwent	-	-	-	11	-	2	2	2	-	-	49	5	5	2	-	10	1	-	2	-
Islwyn	-	-	-	48	-	6	4	4	1	1	13	1	1	-	1	44	21	1	25	-
Monmouth	-	-	-	4	1	-	-	-	-	-	11	1	2	1	1	14	2	-	4	-
Newport	1	-	-	26	-	8	7	7	-	1	113	28	14	6	7	44	43	13	31	1
Torfaen	-	-	-	7	-	4	3	2	-	1	9	2	12	6	1	8	1	19	-	-
Gwynedd	-	-	2	141	-	26	19	19	2	5	158	9	10	3	1	20	39	3	25	3
Aberconwy	-	-	2	27	-	5	5	5	-	-	20	-	4	2	-	4	1	-	1	1
Arfon	-	-	-	11	-	11	8	8	-	3	58	3	3	-	-	1	1	1	-	-
Dwyfor	-	-	-	13	-	3	2	2	-	1	9	3	1	1	-	2	2	1	-	-
Meirionnydd	-	-	-	43	-	4	1	1	2	1	34	-	-	-	-	3	12	1	1	2
Ynys Mon (Anglesey)	-	-	-	47	-	3	3	3	-	-	37	3	2	-	1	10	23	-	23	-
Mid Glamorgan	-	1	39	382	38	22	18	18	-	4	201	18	24	13	2	221	67	45	51	3
Cynon Valley	-	1	2	48	-	4	4	4	-	-	35	1	1	1	-	19	2	-	-	-
Merthyr Tydfil	-	-	-	14	12	7	4	4	-	3	13	-	2	1	-	9	1	7	-	-
Ogwr	-	-	1	182	-	3	2	2	-	1	54	5	8	4	2	30	10	22	16	3
Rhondda	-	-	1	34	2	-	-	-	-	-	23	8	3	1	-	92	20	1	16	-
Rhymney Valley	-	-	30	65	13	5	5	5	-	-	17	1	4	-	-	40	13	10	2	-
Taff-Ely	-	-	5	39	11	3	3	3	-	-	59	3	6	6	-	31	21	5	17	-
Powys	-	-	-	76	1	3	1	1	-	2	15	1	2	1	-	5	6	9	2	1
Brecknock	-	-	-	53	-	2	-	-	-	2	2	-	1	1	-	-	-	1	-	-
Montgomeryshire	-	-	-	23	1	1	1	1	-	-	13	1	1	-	-	5	6	8	2	1
Radnor	-	-	-	-	-	-	-	-	-	-	-	-	-	-	-	-	-	-	-	-
South Glamorgan	-	-	166	518	174	36	29	28	-	7	210	53	29	5	2	89	146	103	33	7
Cardiff	-	-	151	439	174	25	18	18	-	7	162	36	22	4	2	70	82	99	26	6
Vale of Glamorgan	-	-	15	79	-	11	11	10	-	-	48	17	7	1	-	19	64	4	7	1
West Glamorgan	-	-	13	469	134	27	26	23	-	1	145	27	21	6	4	39	24	36	1	5
Lliw Valley	-	-	11	101	1	3	2	2	-	1	23	1	2	1	1	5	-	1	-	-
Neath	-	-	-	76	-	4	4	4	-	-	32	1	1	-	-	2	-	3	-	-
Port Talbot	-	-	-	46	-	6	6	4	-	-	34	6	-	-	1	5	3	6	-	-
Swansea	-	-	2	246	133	14	14	13	-	-	56	19	18	5	2	27	21	26	1	5
Port Health Authorities	1	-	-	-	-	-	-	-	-	-	-	-	-	-	-	1	-	-	-	-

† Categories overlap and therefore some cases will be included in more than one column.
≠ See note on page vi.

Table 5 - *continued*   **Notifications of infectious diseases not shown in main table**

Number of cases and administrative area	Number of cases and administrative area	Number of cases and administrative area	Number of cases and administrative area
9 Tetanus	**20 Leptospirosis** - *continued*	**19 Cholera** - *continued*	**4 Typhus fever** - *continued*
1 Sunderland (Tyne and Wear)	1 Torridge (Devon)	1 Reading (Berks)	1 Southwark (Gtr London)
1 Dartford (Kent)	1 Dudley (W Mids)	1 Wycombe (Bucks)	1 Liverpool (Merseyside)
2 Thanet (Kent)	1 Worcester (Hereford & Worcester)	1 Woodspring (Avon)	
1 Kingston upon Thames	2 St Helens (Merseyside)	1 Worcester (Hereford & Worcester)	**2 Relapsing fever**
(Gtr London)	1 Wirral (Merseyside)	1 Stafford (Staffs)	
1 Cherwell (Oxfordshire)	1 Carmarthen (Dyfed)	1 Ellesmere Port & Neston (Cheshire)	1 Kensington & Chelsea
1 Teignbridge (Devon)		1 Stockport (Gtr Manchester)	(Gtr London)
1 Cotswold (Gloucestershire)	**1 Acute poliomyelitis**	1 Blackpool (Lancs)	1 Dudley (W Mids)
1 St. Helens (Merseyside)		1 Rossendale (Lancs)	
	- Paralytic		**2 Viral haemorrhagic fever**
20 Leptospirosis		**2 Anthrax**	
	1 Manchester (Gtr Manchester)		2 Bromley (Gtr London)
1 Carlisle (Cumbria)		1 Amber Valley (Derbyshire)	
1 Leeds (W Yorks)	**19 Cholera**	1 East Cambridgeshire (Cambs)	
1 E Yorks Boro of Beverley			
(Humberside)	1 Derby (Derbyshire)	**2 Diphtheria**	
1 Craven (N Yorks)	1 Gedling (Notts)		
1 North Kesteven (Lincs)	1 Nottingham (Notts)	1 Hammersmith & Fulham (Gtr London)	
1 St Edmundsbury (Suffolk)	1 Babergh (Suffolk)	1 Rochdale (Gtr Manchester)	
2 Waveney (Suffolk)	1 Chelmsford (Essex)		
1 Bexley (Gtr London)	1 Greenwich (Gtr London)	**4 Typhus fever**	
1 Rother (E Sussex)	1 Lewisham (Gtr London)		
1 Tonbridge & Malling (Kent)	1 Wandsworth (Gtr London)	1 South Tyneside (Tyne & Wear)	
1 Wycombe (Bucks)	1 Crawley (W Sussex)	1 Westminster, city of (Gtr London)	
1 Teignbridge (Devon)	1 Horsham (W Sussex)		

There were no cases of Plague, Smallpox, Yellow fever, or Rabies.

Table 6 Series MB2 no.17

**Table 6 Notifications and deaths assigned to
a few uncommon infectious diseases, 1990**   **England and Wales**

ICD number	Disease	Notifications				Deaths		
		Area	Original	Final		Area	Number	
				M	F		M	F
001	Cholera	Derby	1	-	1		-	-
		Gedling	1	1	-		-	-
		Nottingham	1	-	1		-	-
		Babergh	1	-	1		-	-
		Greenwich	1	-	1		-	-
		Lewisham	1	1	-		-	-
		Wandsworth	1	-	1		-	-
		Reading	1	-	1		-	-
		Wycombe	1	1	-		-	-
		Chelmsford	1	1	-		-	-
		Crawley	1	-	1		-	-
		Horsham	1	1	-		-	-
		Woodspring	1	1	-		-	-
		Worcester	1	-	1		-	-
		Stafford	1	1	-		-	-
		Rochdale	1	-	-		-	-
		Stockport	1	1	-		-	-
		Halton	1	1	-		-	-
		Blackpool	1	-	1		-	-
		Rossendale	1	1	-		-	-
020	Plague	-		-	-		-	-
022	Anthrax	Amber Valley	1	1	-		-	-
		East Cambridgeshire	1	1	-		-	-
023	Brucellosis		*Not notifiable*					
030	Leprosy†		9	8	1	Enfield	1	-
032	Diphtheria	Ipswich	1	-	-		-	-
		Hammersmith and Fulham	1	1	-		-	-
		Rochdale	1	-	1		-	-
039	Actinomycotic infections		*Not notifiable*			Lambeth	1	-
045	Acute poliomyelitis*	Manchester	1	1	-	Swansea	1	-
		Torfaen	1	-	-		-	-
050	Smallpox	-		-	-		-	-
060	Yellow fever	-		-	-		-	-
071	Rabies	Newark and Sherwood	1	-	-		-	-
078.7 & 078.8 (pt)	Viral haemorrhagic fever	Bromley	2	2	-		-	-
080-082	Typhus fever	South Tyneside	1	1	-		-	-
		Southwark	1	-	1		-	-
		Westminster, city of	1	1	-		-	-
		Liverpool	1	1	-		-	-
083.0	Q fever		*Not notifiable*			Bury	-	1
087	Relapsing fever	Kensington and Chelsea	1	-	1		-	-
		Dudley	1	1	-		-	-

* Excludes late effects.
† See note on page v.
Deaths from malaria were reported from Birmingham (1); Gloucester (1); Portsmouth (1).

**Table 7 Tuberculosis of the respiratory system*: death rates
per million population, sex and age-group, 1980 to 1990**   **England and Wales**

Year	Age-group All ages	0-4	5-14	15-24	25-34	35-44	45-54	55-64	65-74	75 and over
Males										
1980	21	-	-	-	*1*	7	19	48	86	152
1981	18	-	-	*1*	2	7	12	35	78	139
1982	17	-	-	*0*	*1*	3	17	34	66	135
1983	16	-	-	-	*1*	3	10	31	67	138
1984	17	-	-	*0*	*1*	2	10	33	69	146
1985	17	-	-	*0*	2	3	8	31	63	152
1986	16	*0*	-	*0*	*0*	2	9	30	68	135
1987	14	-	-	*0*	*1*	*1*	8	25	51	121
1988	17	-	-	*0*	-	3	7	27	71	148
1989	13	-	-	*0*	*1*	4	4	24	49	111
1990	13	*1*	*0*	-	*1*	2	7	20	58	109
Females										
1980	9	-	-	*0*	*1*	3	11	21	23	40
1981	7	-	-	*1*	*1*	*1*	4	14	23	28
1982	8	-	-	*0*	*1*	*1*	9	20	20	37
1983	7	-	*0*	-	*0*	*1*	7	15	24	29
1984	8	-	-	*0*	*0*	2	4	16	26	38
1985	10	-	-	*1*	*1*	*1*	3	19	33	44
1986	9	*1*	*0*	-	*1*	*1*	4	14	26	48
1987	7	-	-	*1*	*1*	*1*	4	16	24	29
1988	8	-	-	*1*	-	*1*	*1*	9	28	40
1989	8	-	-	*0*	*1*	*0*	4	12	30	42
1990	6	-	-	*1*	*1*	*1*	2	10	22	31

* Includes late effects of all tuberculosis (ICD 137)

**Table 8 Tuberculosis† of the respiratory system: notification rates
per 100,000 population, sex and age-group, 1980 to 1990**   **England and Wales**

Year	Age-group All ages	0-4	5-14	15-24	25-34	35-44	45-54	55-64	65-74	75 and over
Males										
1980	17	7	7	14	16	15	20	28	30	36
1981	15	7	5	9	15	13	19	24	27	31
1982	15	5	4	10	15	12	19	23	26	34
1983	13	6	4	8	13	12	15	20	26	33
1984	12	6	3	7	12	9	14	18	25	30
1985	11	4	3	7	10	8	13	17	24	31
1986	11	3	4	6	11	9	12	17	23	30
1987	10	4	3	5	10	9	11	14	19	25
1988	10	2	3	5	10	8	12	14	20	27
1989	10	2	3	6	10	8	11	14	19	27
1990	9	3	3	6	8	8	10	13	18	24
Females										
1980	10	7	6	14	12	10	11	9	8	8
1981	9	5	5	11	11	9	9	9	9	7
1982	9	5	5	11	12	7	9	8	9	11
1983	8	4	4	9	12	7	9	8	9	9
1984	8	6	4	8	10	7	8	9	8	9
1985	8	4	3	8	10	6	7	8	9	10
1986	8	4	4	8	11	7	7	8	10	8
1987	6	3	4	7	8	5	6	7	7	7
1988	6	3	3	7	9	5	5	6	7	8
1989	7	4	4	7	9	5	6	8	7	8
1990	6	3	3	6	8	6	6	8	7	8

† See note on page vi.

Table 9 Tuberculosis of the respiratory system*:
death rates per million population, sex and age-group,
Standardised Mortality Ratios (SMRs), 1990

England and Wales,
standard regions,
regional health authorities

Area	Persons	Males								Females							
	All ages	All ages	0-4	5-14	15-24	25-44	45-64	65 and over	SMR	All ages	0-4	5-14	15-24	25-44	45-64	65 and over	SMR
England and Wales† (excluding port health districts)	10	13	*1*	*0*	-	*1*	13	77	100	6	-	-	*1*	*1*	6	27	100
Wales	15	20	-	-	-	2	*10*	125	143	9	-	-	-	-	*12*	35	*141*
Standard regions																	
North	10	15	-	-	-	2	*12*	*88*	109	6	-	-	-	-	-	*31*	89
Yorkshire and Humberside	8	10	-	-	-	-	*9*	*65*	78	6	-	-	-	*1*	4	28	99
East Midlands	10	16	-	-	-	3	*14*	*94*	121	4	-	-	-	-	2	19	63
East Anglia	6	8	-	-	-	-	*9*	*41*	55	4	-	-	-	-	-	20	58
South East	10	13	-	*1*	-	*1*	15	*76*	101	6	-	-	*1*	*0*	6	27	101
South West	9	12	-	-	-	-	*10*	*67*	82	7	-	-	-	-	4	27	93
West Midlands	12	14	-	-	-	*1*	17	*78*	107	9	-	-	*3*	*3*	*12*	32	153
North West	9	13	*5*	-	-	3	*13*	*71*	100	5	-	-	-	-	9	20	86
Regional health authorities																	
Northern	10	15	-	-	-	2	*12*	*88*	109	6	-	-	-	-	-	*31*	89
Yorkshire	7	7	-	-	-	-	*10*	*40*	55	7	-	-	-	2	5	29	108
Trent	10	18	-	-	-	*1*	*14*	110	132	3	-	-	-	-	-	*19*	53
East Anglian	6	8	-	-	-	-	*9*	*41*	55	4	-	-	-	-	-	20	58
North West Thames	10	12	-	-	-	2	*8*	*79*	93	9	-	-	-	-	*11*	40	151
North East Thames	9	15	-	-	-	2	23	*77*	116	4	-	-	-	-	5	17	66
South East Thames	10	16	-	-	-	-	29	*69*	112	5	-	-	-	-	5	18	69
South West Thames	11	15	-	*6*	-	-	*3*	109	115	8	-	-	*5*	*2*	6	26	*115*
Wessex	8	*10*	-	-	-	-	16	*44*	68	6	-	-	-	-	3	26	87
Oxford	9	*9*	-	-	-	3	*4*	*70*	80	8	-	-	-	-	8	40	140
South Western	10	13	-	-	-	-	*6*	*75*	84	7	-	-	-	-	3	*31*	100
West Midlands	12	14	-	-	-	*1*	17	*78*	107	9	-	-	*3*	*3*	*12*	32	153
Mersey	8	*9*	-	-	-	6	*8*	*42*	66	7	-	-	-	-	*11*	27	*115*
North Western	10	15	*7*	-	-	2	17	*87*	119	4	-	-	-	-	7	*16*	*68*

* Includes late effects of all tuberculosis (ICD 137).
† Deaths of persons normally resident outside England and Wales are included in the England and Wales figures but excluded elsewhere.

Table 10 Tuberculosis of the respiratory system: notification rates
per 100,000 population, sex and age-group, notifications per
100 deaths, Standardised Notification Ratios (SNRs), 1990

England and Wales,
standard regions

Area	Persons	Males								Females								Notification ratio
	All ages	All ages	0-4	5-14	15-24	25-44	45-64	65 and over	SNR	All ages	0-4	5-14	15-24	25-44	45-64	65 and over	SNR	
England and Wales (excluding port health districts)	8	9	3	3	6	8	11	21	100	6	3	3	6	7	7	7	100	**788**
Wales	6	8	-	*1*	3	5	11	24	86	4	*3*	2	*1*	2	3	9	57	388
Standard regions																		
North	6	7	*1*	2	-	5	9	23	76	4	-	2	2	2	7	7	65	548
Yorkshire and Humberside	8	10	2	4	6	7	12	25	106	6	4	2	8	7	6	8	102	971
East Midlands	8	9	*1*	2	6	8	9	24	98	8	4	3	9	9	7	8	119	828
East Anglia	4	4	-	-	3	3	6	*10*	45	3	2	2	3	3	4	4	47	608
South East	9	11	3	2	7	12	14	18	116	8	2	3	6	10	8	8	119	935
South West	3	4	-	0	*1*	3	4	14	45	2	*1*	-	*1*	2	2	4	29	318
West Midlands	10	11	4	5	10	8	13	27	122	8	4	3	10	7	11	10	134	838
North West	9	11	5	5	6	8	14	23	113	7	7	4	8	7	7	8	113	978

Table 11 Deaths with mention of tetanus: sex and age, 1990 **England and Wales**

Age	Sex	Circumstances relating to death, where stated
		(a) assigned to tetanus (ICD 037)
90 years	F	Fell onto garden fence and cut forehead
		(b) assigned elsewhere
		Nil

Table 12 Deaths assigned to infectious diseases where encephalitis is a secondary cause: sex and age-group, 1990* **England and Wales**

ICD number	Underlying cause of death		Deaths assigned to infectious disease													
			Total	With encephalitis as a secondary cause												
				All ages	Age-group (years)											
					Under 1	1	2	3	4	5-9	10-14	15-24	25-44	45-64	65 and over
	Total	M	445	18	-	1	-	-	-	-	1	-	9	4	3
		F	122	12	-	-	-	-	1	1	1	1	3	2	3
052	Chicken pox	M	10	1	-	-	-	-	-	-	-	-	-	-	1
		F	14	2	-	-	-	-	1	-	-	-	1	-	-
053	Herpes zoster	M	27	1	-	-	-	-	-	-	-	-	-	-	1
		F	61	1	-	-	-	-	-	-	-	-	-	-	1
054	Herpes simplex	M	13	6	-	1	-	-	-	-	-	-	2	2	1
		F	11	7	-	-	-	-	-	-	1	1	1	2	2
055	Measles	M	1	1	-	-	-	-	-	-	1	-	-	-	-
		F	-	-	-	-	-	-	-	-	-	-	-	-	-
279	Disorders involving the immune mechanism	M	394	9	-	-	-	-	-	-	-	-	7	2	-
		F	36	1	-	-	-	-	-	-	-	-	1	-	-

* From 1986 neonatal deaths by cause are excluded (see note on page 2).

Table 13 Series MB2 no.17

Table 13 Identifications of viruses, chlamydias, rickettsias and mycoplasmas, 1986 to 1989†; 1990 by age

England and Wales*

Organism	1986	1987	1988	1989	1990 All ages	Under 1	1-4	5-9	10-14	15-44	45-64	65 and over	Not stated
Adenovirus	4,210	4,470	4,886	4,170	**4,309**	1,570	1,351	185	75	741	132	48	207
1,2, 5 and 6	1,111	914	1,025	959	**942**	453	335	33	7	55	8	7	44
3	149	476	665	262	**419**	47	98	45	10	159	34	7	19
4	285	434	497	299	**292**	17	16	7	13	172	34	7	26
7	154	145	83	47	**96**	22	25	15	3	24	3	1	3
Coxsackie A	102	378	200	159	**247**	79	59	12	12	63	2	2	18
A9	21	356	134	89	**208**	63	50	12	12	55	1	2	13
A16	48	4	24	36	**11**	1	5	-	-	1	-	-	4
A21	4	3	17	21	**-**	-	-	-	-	-	-	-	-
Coxsackie B	415	551	636	298	**536**	195	181	34	7	75	7	3	34
B2	133	165	58	79	**135**	53	42	5	3	16	-	1	15
B4	47	38	253	51	**-**	-	-	-	-	-	-	-	-
B5	53	34	212	100	**60**	21	21	4	1	10	-	2	1
Cytomegalovirus	1,273	1,166	1,272	1,157	**1,316**	235	71	30	30	440	288	105	117
Echovirus	1,783	1,034	1,445	1,393	**694**	321	140	52	22	124	4	2	29
7	48	8	28	396	**53**	24	14	3	2	8	-	-	2
9	125	350	291	111	**-**	-	-	-	-	-	-	-	-
11	445	79	364	284	**48**	18	15	1	1	10	-	-	3
22	391	285	268	179	**-**	-	-	-	-	-	-	-	-
30	307	111	141	113	**15**	1	2	4	3	4	-	-	1
Hepatitis B antigen	2,771	2,563	2,439	2,242	**1,904**	32	18	16	22	1,335	303	57	121
Herpes simplex	16,995	14,171	13,783	7,587	**10,113**	16	7	4	18	7,602	398	42	2,026
Varicella zoster	564	527	512	530	**312**	11	13	10	5	172	41	39	21
Influenza A	1,959	819	484	1,629	**2,562**	213	195	118	100	452	433	827	224
B	721	190	1,829	43	**345**	17	7	16	36	146	45	64	14
C	1	-	-	-	**1**	1	-	-	-	-	-	-	-
Measles	287	172	310	119	**78**	-	4	11	5	38	9	7	4
Mumps	547	688	428	265	**94**	2	28	11	4	34	5	6	4
Orf-paravaccinia	69	37	32	13	**15**	-	-	-	-	12	1	-	2
Parainfluenza	627	731	578	643	**494**	341	84	13	7	23	5	4	17
Poliovirus	578	495	541	390	**112**	97	3	1	-	3	-	-	8
RS virus	4,443	6,019	8,898	5,057	**7,141**	5,697	675	44	13	60	39	70	543
Rhinovirus	364	418	341	350	**322**	212	37	16	6	29	2	5	15
Rotavirus	8,298	9,120	10,378	13,493	**14,498**	5,879	6,411	305	66	183	84	385	1,185
Rubella	2,037	1,887	1,031	760	**705**	6	32	18	30	543	53	3	20
Vaccinia	-	-	-	-	**-**	-	-	-	-	-	-	-	-
Chlamydia A	29,599	27,870	26,801	26,371	**30,078**	580	13	10	81	21,393	395	44	7,562
B	326	430	460	574	**485**	1	1	2	9	200	179	77	16
Coxiella burnetii	146	160	144	228	**156**	1	2	1	3	69	54	20	6
Mycoplasma pneumoniae	1,696	2,522	864	875	**1,410**	15	104	209	123	654	152	76	77

See notes on page vi.
* The figures include some identifications from Northern Ireland, Eire, Channel Islands and Isle of Man. In **Tables 14** and **15** the number of identifications from this group is shown.
† Laboratory data for 1989 were not verified; comparison with other years is therefore invalid.

Table 14 Identifications of viruses, chlamydias, rickettsias and mycoplasmas, 1990

England and Wales*, regional health authorities

Organism	England and Wales *	Wales	Regional health authorities Northern	Yorkshire	Trent	East Anglian	North West Thames	North East Thames	South East Thames	South West Thames	Wessex	Oxford	South Western	West Midlands	Mersey	North Western	N Ireland, Eire, CI, IOM
Adenovirus	4,309	200	402	294	337	201	90	187	357	87	183	174	456	461	349	391	140
1,2,5 and 6	942	26	172	95	50	64	7	19	16	1	23	10	125	99	88	143	4
3	419	2	54	47	31	27	-	2	7	2	19	18	55	80	21	53	1
4	292	2	23	29	21	12	1	2	2	1	52	2	49	53	16	26	1
7	96	1	5	9	11	3	-	2	3	1	1	2	6	7	8	35	2
Coxsackie A	247	4	31	35	22	10	9	5	8	11	9	10	30	22	11	19	11
A9	208	3	22	34	21	4	7	5	7	6	7	10	27	16	10	19	10
A16	11	-	-	-	-	6	2	-	-	-	-	-	2	1	-	-	-
A21	-	-	-	-	-	-	-	-	-	-	-	-	-	-	-	-	-
Coxsackie B	536	13	105	51	24	7	9	19	13	2	27	16	42	72	68	53	15
B2	135	3	27	9	7	4	2	8	3	1	5	3	12	25	11	6	9
B5	60	-	4	3	-	-	-	4	5	-	4	3	4	18	9	6	-
Cytomegalovirus	1,316	18	91	49	108	96	107	43	92	112	88	75	63	162	21	168	23
Echovirus	694	18	96	92	42	16	24	14	23	14	13	35	61	117	37	35	57
7	53	3	5	4	4	-	-	1	-	1	-	-	6	17	2	2	8
9	-	-	-	-	-	-	-	-	-	-	-	-	-	-	-	-	-
11	48	-	7	9	3	3	3	-	2	-	1	5	3	5	6	-	1
22	-	-	-	-	-	-	-	-	-	-	-	-	-	-	-	-	-
30	15	-	-	-	2	-	1	-	2	1	4	-	-	1	2	2	-
Hepatitis B antigen	1,904	68	63	156	85	46	197	89	290	133	79	26	88	282	139	128	35
Herpes simplex	10,113	206	267	735	1,570	506	914	442	570	601	754	577	943	1,203	302	427	96
Varicella zoster	312	12	21	23	40	24	17	11	16	5	17	15	27	22	16	37	9
Influenza A	2,562	66	122	106	211	279	87	48	235	138	149	76	491	213	133	127	81
B	345	5	37	14	21	65	13	10	21	14	13	11	41	31	16	31	2
C	1	-	-	-	-	-	-	-	-	-	1	-	-	-	-	-	-
Measles	78	11	11	1	7	11	3	-	14	2	-	1	5	4	1	2	5
Mumps	94	10	6	2	10	5	4	1	17	2	7	1	3	5	8	8	5
Orf-paravaccinia	15	1	2	2	2	-	-	-	1	-	1	1	2	2	1	-	-
Parainfluenza	494	31	59	35	26	18	21	19	28	23	28	15	74	48	25	42	2
Poliovirus	112	2	1	17	12	-	1	5	5	-	2	1	10	28	4	20	4
RS virus	7,141	415	696	391	980	296	230	419	288	346	368	260	476	618	380	793	185
Rhinovirus	322	6	159	-	25	12	5	16	11	4	31	17	15	7	7	7	-
Rotavirus	14,498	610	743	2,450	1,264	397	760	1,171	668	577	674	545	1,044	1,787	666	982	160
Rubella	705	28	81	36	42	29	25	15	28	35	33	60	96	60	50	61	26
Vaccinia	-	-	-	-	-	-	-	-	-	-	-	-	-	-	-	-	-
Chlamydia A	30,078	934	2,093	2,218	4,203	818	1,582	1,063	1,847	1,217	722	1,224	2,932	4,961	681	3,222	361
B	485	25	11	14	51	67	5	17	46	14	20	26	89	41	9	16	34
Coxiella burnetii	156	3	1	1	9	6	-	1	4	4	4	4	28	13	9	1	68
Mycoplasma pneumoniae	1,410	49	48	14	68	105	38	43	99	98	94	79	231	126	59	118	141

See notes on page vi.

* The figures include some identifications from Northern Ireland, Eire, Channel Islands and Isle of Man. In this table and **Table 15** the number of identifications from this group is shown.

Table 15 Series MB2 no.17

Table 15 Identifications†≠ of shigellas, salmonellas and Escherichia coli: 1989ψ; 1990 by area

Organism	1989ψ	1990		Regional health authorities					
	England and Wales*	England and Wales*	Wales	Northern	Yorkshire	Trent	East Anglian	North West Thames	North East Thames
Shigellas	**3,556**	**3,405**	355	102	627	140	87	269	178
S. boydii	161	95	3	2	18	1	3	16	6
S. dysenteriae	73	44	1	-	5	3	1	7	2
S. flexneri	774	841	18	13	136	44	20	76	59
S. sonnei	2,548	2,425	333	87	468	92	63	170	111
Salmonellas	**25,342**	**26,203**	1,313	1,715	3,215	2,563	921	1,158	1,435
S. typhi									
cases and excretors††	81	101	-	4	15	11	2	19	8
S. paratyphi A									
cases and excretors††	44	42	2	-	4	1	2	4	5
S. paratyphi B									
cases and excretors††	22	34	1	5	2	-	-	2	2
S. paratyphi C									
cases and excretors††	-	-	-	-	-	-	-	-	-
S. typhimurium	6,188	4,757	252	843	577	426	161	162	220
S. agona	156	158	2	7	19	16	9	5	8
S. anatum	45	83	2	3	14	10	1	8	2
S. bareilly	27	25	-	1	2	1	1	3	2
S. berta	45	99	10	27	6	6	4	4	4
S. blockley	68	90	3	5	7	3	5	3	7
S. bovis-morbificans	56	31	1	2	5	2	2	2	1
S. braenderup	90	100	1	5	12	11	1	6	6
S. brandenburg	66	76	3	1	6	2	1	1	9
S. bredeney	70	90	2	4	6	3	2	3	1
S. derby	66	74	7	3	7	6	2	4	3
S. dublin	65	30	4	-	5	-	-	3	-
S. enteritidis	13,231	16,002	805	564	2,054	1,636	615	729	912
S. give	22	30	-	2	-	5	-	-	2
S. gold-coast	69	24	-	-	1	9	-	-	1
S. hadar	327	236	21	11	26	22	4	7	14
S. heidelberg	288	313	24	18	20	19	5	13	9
S. indiana	51	50	1	1	13	7	1	2	1
S. infantis	326	330	27	32	34	27	10	10	19
S. java	26	31	2	2	5	2	1	2	1
S. javiana	10	23	-	-	4	1	-	1	2
S. kedougou	278	228	3	11	23	13	-	1	5
S. livingstone	38	60	1	8	2	8	1	1	2
S. london	21	21	-	1	1	1	-	1	1
S. mbandaka	48	84	2	6	15	4	1	2	4
S. montevideo	142	211	10	12	19	14	8	9	28
S. muenchen	35	28	-	-	6	2	-	3	-
S. newington	7	22	-	-	4	8	1	-	2
S. newport	313	307	19	16	26	46	8	13	12
S. ohio	78	47	1	2	6	1	-	9	6
S. oranienburg	33	40	1	2	2	4	-	1	3
S. panama	231	160	6	6	37	22	3	9	5
S. portsmouth	1	32	1	1	1	3	1	1	2
S. saint-paul	98	80	2	3	6	5	3	3	5
S. schwarzengrund	36	36	1	-	1	2	1	-	5
S. senftenberg	29	40	5	-	7	2	2	3	4
S. stanley	87	105	3	9	14	5	3	3	3
S. thompson	86	131	5	12	36	4	7	6	3
S. unnamed	76	121	8	2	7	4	2	4	4
S. virchow	1,531	1,083	55	66	82	149	32	63	68
Others	735	538	20	18	76	40	19	33	34
E coli**	**1,448**	**1,323**	**92**	**152**	**216**	**118**	**28**	**46**	**68**

See notes on page vi.
†   Includes cases, carriers and excretors.
*   The figures include some identifications from Northern Ireland, Eire, Channel Islands and Isle of Man. In this table and **Table 14** the number of identifications from this group is shown.
††   Cases not reported directly to CDSC by the source laboratory are not included.
**   Enteropathogenic group in children under 3 years of age with gastroenteritis.
≠   Faecal isolates only.
ψ   Laboratory data for 1989 were not verified; comparison with other years is therefore invalid.

England and Wales*,
regional health authorities

1990ψ									Organism
Regional health authorities								N Ireland, Eire, CI, IOM	
South East Thames	South West Thames	Wessex	Oxford	South Western	West Midlands	Mersey	North Western		
176	**294**	**96**	**161**	**201**	**198**	**28**	**363**	**130**	**Shigellas**
9	12	3	7	4	7	-	4	-	S. boydii
5	2	3	1	2	4	-	8	-	S. dysenteriae
51	102	24	52	47	69	9	103	18	S. flexneri
111	178	66	101	148	118	19	248	112	S. sonnei
1,298	**1,496**	**1,845**	**1,342**	**1,900**	**2,430**	**810**	**2,210**	**552**	**Salmonellas**
									S. typhi
4	12	-	3	1	12	-	10	-	*cases and excretors††*
									S. paratyphi A
1	4	-	3	3	7	-	5	1	*cases and excretors††*
									S. paratyphi B
1	2	7	3	2	-	1	6	-	*cases and excretors††*
									S. paratyphi C
-	-	-	-	-	-	-	-	-	*cases and excretors††*
229	205	322	193	273	430	114	255	95	S. typhimurium
4	13	8	6	6	15	6	26	8	S. agona
3	7	8	4	4	9	-	8	-	S. anatum
-	4	-	2	-	2	1	6	-	S. bareilly
1	6	7	3	6	4	4	6	1	S. berta
8	7	4	5	6	9	9	9	-	S. blockley
1	2	2	2	3	1	-	5	-	S. bovis-morbificans
4	15	6	4	9	8	4	8	-	S. braenderup
3	4	4	1	4	5	13	17	2	S. brandenburg
3	2	4	5	2	2	1	2	48	S. bredeney
4	4	6	5	3	6	1	13	-	S. derby
-	5	1	4	5	3	-	-	-	S. dublin
817	930	1,211	843	1,283	1,512	492	1,260	339	S. enteritidis
3	3	2	2	4	4	1	2	-	S. give
1	1	3	1	-	3	1	-	3	S. gold-coast
17	12	10	14	21	16	16	23	2	S. hadar
14	11	22	18	19	92	7	19	3	S. heidelberg
2	3	1	1	5	3	2	7	-	S. indiana
23	25	25	11	24	26	6	27	4	S. infantis
1	1	1	1	4	3	-	3	2	S. java
1	2	1	4	4	3	-	-	-	S. javiana
2	-	3	2	-	9	13	143	-	S. kedougou
3	3	17	2	2	4	3	3	-	S. livingstone
2	1	5	-	5	1	-	2	-	S. london
2	2	4	9	3	8	1	21	-	S. mbandaka
12	19	7	21	13	16	11	11	1	S. montevideo
4	1	-	2	5	-	1	2	2	S. muenchen
-	1	1	-	-	-	-	5	-	S. newington
12	20	13	11	8	38	11	48	6	S. newport
2	1	5	1	2	6	2	2	1	S. ohio
5	3	2	3	3	4	2	4	1	S. oranienburg
7	8	4	8	9	21	3	12	-	S. panama
-	-	-	-	-	3	1	18	-	S. portsmouth
3	4	12	6	9	12	2	2	3	S. saint-paul
2	-	-	1	1	1	3	18	-	S. schwarzengrund
-	3	2	2	5	4	-	1	-	S. senftenberg
2	7	6	1	2	9	5	33	-	S. stanley
9	5	4	10	11	5	2	12	-	S. thompson
5	8	5	2	11	12	26	19	2	S. unnamed
48	84	64	77	76	63	32	106	18	S. virchow
33	46	36	46	44	39	13	31	10	Others
49	**40**	**31**	**12**	**73**	**94**	**14**	**144**	**146**	**E coli****

Table 16 Series MB2 no.17

Table 16 Identifications of various organisms including helminths and protozoa: 1989†; 1990 by age England and Wales*

Organism/syndrome	1989	1990 All ages	Under 1	1-4	5-9	10-14	15-44	45-64	65 and over	Not stated
Bacteria										
Actinomycosis	64	53	-	-	-	-	33	14	4	2
Bacillus anthracis	-	-	-	-	-	-	-	-	-	-
Bordetella	719	1,004	see below							
Brucella†	17	10	-	-	-	-	5	2	1	2
Clostridium tetani	3	1	-	-	-	-	-	-	1	-
Corynebacterium diphtheriae toxigenic	6	3	-	1	1	-	1	-	-	-
Leptospira**	55	28	-	-	-	-	21	6	1	-
Mycobacterium										
bovis	22	13	-	-	-	-	1	4	6	2
tuberculosis (non-resp)	560	452	1	3	6	6	196	117	94	29
other	224	256	-	13	11	3	63	64	78	24
Neisseria meningitidis (CSF/blood only)	1,061	1,223	289	312	83	59	344	65	48	23
Vibrio cholerae	1	6	-	2	-	-	4	-	-	-
Helminths										
Schistosoma**	96	97	-	-	4	3	39	2	-	49
Echinococcus	25	14	-	-	-	-	2	4	2	6
Taenia	69	84	-	1	3	2	45	11	1	21
Ascaris	730	287	1	22	67	44	76	15	3	59
Strongyloides	67	56	-	4	1	-	19	12	1	19
Trichuris	566	588	3	35	114	96	167	39	7	127
Hookworms, unspecified	458	457	-	10	46	57	169	45	12	118
Filaria										
Loa Loa	7	6	-	-	-	-	1	-	-	5
Onchocerca volvulus	4	15	-	-	-	-	-	-	-	15
Wuchereria bancrofti	2	-	-	-	-	-	-	-	-	-
Dipetalonema perstans	2	5	-	-	-	-	-	-	-	5
Unspecified	1	1	-	-	1	-	-	-	-	-
Protozoa										
Entamoeba histolytica	809	815	3	10	20	17	217	50	18	480
Giardia	6,423	7,064	see below							
Plasmodium										
falciparum	155	161	-	11	8	8	99	25	5	5
malariae	3	7	-	-	-	2	4	-	-	1
ovale	6	23	-	-	-	2	20	-	-	1
vivax	225	255	3	20	16	20	118	44	23	11
Toxoplasma gondii**	955	726	13	6	16	28	471	88	25	79

	1990 Bordetella		1990 Giardia
Total	**1,004**	**Total**	**7,064**
Under 6 months	304	Under 5 years	1,511
6-11 months	77	5-9 years	641
1-5 years	377	10-14 years	296
6 years and over	204	15-24 years	743
Not stated	42	25 years and over	3,024
		Not stated	849

See notes on page vi.
† Laboratory data for 1989 were not verified; comparison with other years is therefore invalid.
* The figures include some identifications from Northern Ireland, Eire, Channel Islands and Isle of Man. In **Tables 14** and **15** the number of identifications from this group is shown.
** Includes cases identified by serology.

Table 17 Organisms associated with* meningitis and/or encephalitis: 1989†; 1990 by age

England and Wales**

Organism	1989†	1990	Age-groups							
		All ages	Under 1	1-4	5-9	10-14	15-44	45-64	65 and over	Not stated
Viruses										
Adenovirus	2	**3**	-	-	2	-	1	-	-	-
Coxsackie A	25	**63**	7	3	5	6	33	1	-	8
B	19	**45**	14	5	3	1	18	-	-	4
Echovirus	196	**106**	13	8	11	9	54	4	-	7
Herpes simplex	10	**17**	3	2	-	-	2	6	2	2
Varicella zoster	4	**1**	-	-	-	-	-	1	-	-
Influenza A	-	**1**	-	-	-	1	-	-	-	-
B	-	**-**	-	-	-	-	-	-	-	-
Measles	10	**10**	-	-	9	1	-	-	-	-
Mumps	14	**11**	-	9	-	-	1	-	-	1
Other viruses	5	**7**	-	1	-	-	3	3	-	-
Mycoplasma pneumoniae	1	**2**	-	-	1	1	-	-	-	-
Bacteria (CSF only)										
Escherichia coli	68	**78**	55	1	1	-	1	11	5	4
Haemophilus influenzae	642	**791**	331	368	27	3	14	19	8	21
Listeria monocytogenes	46	**29**	6	-	-	-	1	10	12	-
Neisseria meningitidis	803	**1,299**	319	336	89	72	376	60	22	25
Staphylococcus aureus	50	**85**	16	6	3	5	12	18	23	2
S. epidermidis	40	**37**	10	4	2	1	8	8	3	1
Streptococcus pneumoniae	389	**578**	138	79	15	10	92	109	107	28
Streptococcus other	124	**179**	106	9	5	4	15	14	16	10
Other bacteria	96	**158**	47	12	6	5	33	33	14	8

See notes on page vi.
* Causal association not necessarily implied.
** The figures include some identifications from Northern Ireland, Eire, Channel Islands and Isle of Man. In **Tables 14** and **15** the number of identifications from this group is shown.
† Laboratory data for 1989 were not verified; comparison with other years is therefore invalid.

Table 18 Series MB2 no.17

Table 18   Newly diagnosed episodes of communicable and respiratory diseases: annual and quarterly totals and rates per 100,000 population at risk, 1988 to 1990

ICD number	Disease	Numbers							
		1988†	1989	1990	13 - week period ended				
					2.1.90	3.4.90	3.7.90	2.10.90	1.1.91
	Communicable diseases								
	Total	**52,056**	**61,060**	**62,620**	**16,989**	**16,433**	**15,257**	**14,301**	**16,629**
003-005, 007-009, 787.0(pt)	Intestinal infectious disease	11,547	13,577	13,889	3,287	3,267	3,263	3,493	3,866
033	Whooping cough	89	183	236	59	56	59	64	57
034	Scarlet fever	338	480	473	127	198	118	74	83
	Meningitis/encephalitis	24	21	23	2	3	6	4	10
052	Chicken pox	2,177	2,683	2,229	313	510	682	524	513
053	Herpes zoster	1,122	1,289	1,342	297	324	343	352	323
055	Measles	912	222	154	41	55	30	34	35
056	Rubella	743	553	384	73	118	135	84	47
070	Infective hepatitis	67	109	96	18	26	26	21	23
072	Mumps	781	590	220	70	84	52	40	44
075	Infective mononucleosis	391	369	381	96	131	86	76	88
133.0	Scabies	563	634	688	186	211	139	149	189
382.9(pt)	Acute otitis media	14,312	15,485	16,290	5,554	5,029	3,592	2,780	4,889
	Other recognised communicable diseases not included above	18,990	24,865	26,215	6,866	6,421	6,726	6,606	6,462
	Respiratory diseases								
	Total	**112,378**	**126,548**	**126,927**	**47,387**	**36,217**	**29,992**	**22,844**	**37,944**
460(pt)	Common cold	41,134	45,460	48,009	16,355	13,216	11,513	8,540	14,740
460(rem)	Influenza-like illnesses	7,505	7,703	4,316	4,430	1,292	963	751	1,310
461	Acute sinusitis	7,084	7,463	8.818	2,278	2,799	2,047	1,482	2,490
462,463	Sore throat, tonsilitis	15,819	17,504	18,081	4,751	5,304	4,499	3,648	4,630
464	Laryngitis and tracheitis	4,792	5,391	4,883	1,938	1,442	1,124	835	1,482
466(pt)	Acute bronchitis	22,653	25,627	27,653	10,239	7,737	6,130	4,663	9,123
480-486	Pneumonia and pneumonitis	702	762	647	321	197	147	119	184
487	Epidemic influenza	2,497	4,472	1,290	3,527	696	124	88	382
493	Acute asthmatic episode	6,071	6,777	7,823	1,936	2,003	2,025	1,673	2,122
511	Pleurisy	323	395	487	146	133	108	94	152
	Other diseases of respiratory system not included above	3,798	4,994	4,920	1,466	1,398	1,242	951	1,329
	Average number of general practices	56	60	62	62	60	58	64	66
	Approximate population at risk	344,000	383,000	404,000	390,000	398,000	396,000	405,000	415,000

See notes on page vi.
* Includes 1 practice in Scotland and 1 practice in Northern Ireland.
† 1988 = 53 weeks (figures include week ending 3 January 1989).

England and Wales*
(Figures derived from returns submitted to the Birmingham Research Unit of the Royal College of General Practitioners)

Rates per 100,000 population								Disease	ICD number
1988†	1989	1990	13-week period ended						
			2.1.90	3.4.90	3.7.90	2.10.90	1.1.91		
								Communicable diseases	
15,147.5	15,921.9	15,518.5	4,359.3	4,124.6	3,854.3	3,534.5	4,005.1	Total	
3,360.0	3,540.3	3,442.0	843.4	820.0	824.3	863.3	931.1	Intestinal infectious disease	003-005, 007-009, 787.0(pt)
25.9	47.7	58.5	15.1	14.1	14.9	15.8	13.7	Whooping cough	033
98.4	125.2	117.2	32.6	49.7	29.8	18.3	20.0	Scarlet fever	034
7.0	5.5	5.7	0.5	0.7	1.5	1.0	2.4	Meningitis/encephalitis	
633.5	699.6	552.4	80.3	128.0	172.3	129.5	123.6	Chicken pox	052
326.5	336.1	332.6	76.2	81.3	86.7	87.0	77.8	Herpes zoster	053
265.4	57.9	38.2	10.5	13.8	7.6	8.4	8.4	Measles	055
216.2	144.2	95.2	18.7	29.6	34.1	20.8	11.3	Rubella	056
19.5	28.4	23.8	4.6	6.5	6.6	5.2	5.5	Infective hepatitis	070
227.3	153.8	54.5	18.0	21.1	13.1	9.9	10.6	Mumps	072
113.8	96.2	94.4	24.6	32.9	21.7	18.8	21.2	Infective mononucleosis	075
163.8	165.3	170.5	47.7	52.9	35.1	36.8	45.5	Scabies	133.0
4,164.6	4,037.8	4,037.0	1,425.1	1,262.2	907.4	687.1	1,177.5	Acute otitis media	382.9(pt)
5,525.8	6,483.7	6,496.6	1,761.8	1,611.6	1,699.2	1,632.7	1,556.4	Other recognised communicable diseases not included above	
								Respiratory diseases	
32,700.2	32,998.3	31,455.2	12,159.3	9,090.2	7,559.1	5,645.8	9,138.9	Total	
11,969.4	11,854.0	11,897.6	4,196.6	3,317.1	2,908.5	2,110.6	3,550.1	Common cold	460(pt)
2,183.8	2,008.6	1,069.6	1,136.7	324.3	243.3	185.6	315.5	Influenza-like illnesses	460(rem)
2,061.3	1,946.0	2,185.3	584.5	702.5	517.1	366.3	599.7	Acute sinusitis	461
4,603.1	4,564.3	4,480.9	1,219.1	1,331.3	1,136.6	901.6	1,115.1	Sore throat, tonsillitis	462,463
1,394.4	1,405.7	1,210.1	497.3	361.9	283.9	206.4	356.9	Laryngitis and tracheitis	464
6,591.7	6,682.4	6,853.0	2,627.3	1,941.9	1,548.6	1,152.4	2,197.3	Acute bronchitis	466(pt)
204.3	198.7	160.3	82.4	49.4	37.1	29.4	44.3	Pneumonia and pneumonitis	480-486
726.6	1,166.1	319.7	905.0	174.7	31.3	21.7	92.0	Epidemic influenza	487
1,766.6	1,767.2	1,938.7	496.8	502.7	511.6	413.5	511.1	Acute asthmatic episode	493
94.0	103.0	120.7	37.5	33.4	27.3	23.2	36.6	Pleurisy	511
1,105.2	1,302.2	1,219.3	376.2	350.9	313.8	235.0	320.1	Other diseases of respiratory system not included above	
56	60	62	62	60	58	64	66	Average number of general practices	
344,000	383,000	404,000	390,000	398,000	396,000	405,000	415,000	Approximate population at risk	

Table 19 Series MB2 no.17

Table 19 Air temperature, rainfall and sunshine: district, 1990

Districts of England and Wales
(Supplied by the Chief Executive)
of the Meteorological Office)

Period	Districts	Air temperature (°C)			Rainfall*		Sunshine*
		Highest maximum	Lowest minimum	Difference from average* daily mean	Percentage of average	Number of rain days† difference from average	Percentage of average
March quarter	England East and North East	21.0	- 4.8	+ 3.3	122	+ 1	122
	East Anglia	21.9	- 3.7	+ 3.4	112	- 2	140
	Midland Counties	21.7	- 6.6	+ 3.3	126	+ 1	132
	England South East and Central Southern	22.0	- 2.3	+ 3.4	140	0	122
	England North West and North Wales	20.2	- 3.0	+ 2.9	159	+ 2	95
	England South West and South Wales	19.5	- 4.7	+ 2.9	140	+ 2	93
	Mean			**+ 3.2**	**133**	**+ 1**	**117**
June quarter	England East and North East	26.0	- 6.0	+ 0.3	78	- 1	109
	East Anglia	26.2	- 6.2	+ 0.4	71	- 3	119
	Midland Counties	28.3	- 6.6	+ 0.4	64	- 3	111
	England South East and Central Southern	28.1	- 4.8	+ 0.5	70	- 3	120
	England North West and North Wales	27.0	- 5.0	+ 0.5	84	+ 1	103
	England South West and South Wales	26.7	- 5.5	+ 0.6	75	0	109
	Mean			**+ 0.5**	**74**	**- 2**	**112**
September quarter	England East and North East	34.8	- 0.2	+ 0.9	59	- 3	124
	East Anglia	35.6	+ 0.2	+ 1.0	49	- 4	126
	Midland Counties	37.1	+ 0.3	+ 1.2	50	- 4	132
	England South East and Central Southern	36.5	+ 3.5	+ 1.2	42	- 5	133
	England North West and North Wales	35.2	+ 1.6	+ 0.7	65	- 3	121
	England South West and South Wales	34.9	+ 0.5	+ 1.1	65	- 3	131
	Mean			**+ 1.0**	**55**	**- 4**	**128**
December quarter	England East and North East	22.9	- 4.0	+ 0.9	109	+ 1	88
	East Anglia	24.5	- 3.0	+ 0.7	91	+ 1	100
	Midland Counties	24.0	- 6.0	+ 0.6	105	0	97
	England South East and Central Southern	24.2	- 5.4	+ 0.6	90	- 1	112
	England North West and North Wales	24.3	- 4.4	+ 0.3	113	- 1	97
	England South West and South Wales	22.0	- 5.5	+ 0.2	96	- 1	112
	Mean			**+ 0.6**	**101**	**- 1**	**101**
Year 1990	England East and North East	34.8	- 6.0	+ 1.4	93	- 5	112
	East Anglia	35.6	- 6.2	+ 1.4	79	-23	120
	Midland Counties	37.1	- 6.6	+ 1.4	85	-17	119
	England South East and Central Southern	36.5	- 5.4	+ 1.4	85	-23	123
	England North West and North Wales	35.2	- 4.4	+ 1.2	106	+ 4	106
	England South West and South Wales	34.9	- 5.5	+ 1.2	96	+12	114
	Mean			**+ 1.3**	**91**	**- 9**	**116**

* 1941-70 averages.

† A rain day is a period of 24 hours commencing at 0900 GMT, on which 0.2 mm (0.01 inch) or more of rainfall is recorded.

Table 20 Air temperature, rainfall and sunshine, 1931 to 1990

England and Wales
(Supplied by the Chief Executive)
of the Meteorological Office)

Year	Air temperature (° C)		Rainfall (mm)		Daily sunshine (hours)	
	Daily mean	Departure from average*	Actual	Departure from average*	Mean	Departure from average*
1931	9.6	-0.5	975	+ 71	3.60	- 0.37
1932	9.9	-0.2	922	+ 18	3.53	- 0.44
1933	10.3	+0.2	726	- 178	4.42	+0.45
1934	10.5	+0.4	851	- 53	4.08	+0.11
1935	10.3	+0.2	1,011	+107	4.13	+0.16
1936	9.9	-0.2	975	+ 71	3.56	- 0.41
1937	10.1	0.0	986	+ 82	3.46	- 0.51
1938	10.6	+0.5	886	+ 18	3.84	- 0.13
1939	10.2	+0.1	1,013	+109	3.97	0.00
1940	9.6	-0.5	904	0	4.18	+0.21
1941	9.6	-0.5	859	- 45	3.67	- 0.30
1942	9.6	-0.5	841	- 63	3.90	- 0.07
1943	10.6	+0.5	833	- 71	4.25	+0.28
1944	10.1	0.0	897	- 7	3.73	- 0.24
1945	10.8	+0.7	833	- 71	3.81	- 0.16
1946	10.0	-0.1	1,057	+153	3.83	- 0.14
1947	10.1	0.0	823	- 81	3.97	0.00
1948	10.5	+0.4	953	+ 49	4.12	+0.15
1949	11.1	+1.0	785	- 119	4.63	+0.66
1950	10.1	0.0	1,021	+117	3.94	- 0.02
1951	9.8	-0.3	1,110	+206	3.98	+0.02
1952	9.7	-0.4	902	- 2	4.10	+0.14
1953	10.4	+0.3	757	- 147	4.04	+0.08
1954	9.8	-0.3	1,085	+181	3.52	0.44
1955	9.8	-0.3	785	- 119	4.47	+0.51
1956	9.4	-0.7	869	- 35	3.88	- 0.08
1957	10.6	+0.5	899	- 5	4.04	+0.08
1958	9.9	-0.2	1,029	- 125	3.52	- 0.44
1959	10.9	+0.8	805	- 99	4.67	+0.71
1960	10.2	+0.1	1,171	+267	3.84	- 0.12
1961	10.5	+0.4	881	- 23	4.12	+0.16
1962	9.2	-0.9	790	- 114	4.16	+0.20
1963	9.0	-1.2	851	- 53	3.87	- 0.08
1964	10.1	-0.1	706	- 198	3.83	- 0.12
1965	9.5	-0.7	996	+ 92	3.67	- 0.28
1966	10.1	-0.1	1,030	+126	3.63	- 0.32
1967	10.3	+0.1	983	+ 79	4.11	+0.16
1968	10.0	-0.2	979	+ 75	3.48	- 0.47
1969	9.9	-0.3	913	+ 9	3.79	- 0.16
1970	10.1	-0.1	910	+ 6	4.07	+0.12
1971	10.4	+0.2	800	- 104	4.03	+0.08
1972	9.8	-0.4	848	- 56	3.67	- 0.28
1973	10.2	0.0	738	- 166	4.11	+0.16
1974	10.0	0.0	994	+ 90	4.08	+0.04
1975	10.4	+0.4	753	- 151	4.36	+0.32
1976	10.5	+0.5	794	- 110	4.40	+0.36
1977	10.0	0.0	925	+ 13	3.95	- 0.09
1978	9.8	-0.2	903	- 9	3.65	- 0.39
1979	8.6	-0.8	1,001	+ 89	3.51	- 0.53
1980	9.9	-0.1	976	+ 64	3.88	- 0.16
1981	9.7	-0.3	999	+ 87	3.64	- 0.40
1982	10.4	+0.4	973	+ 61	4.09	+0.05
1983	10.5	+0.5	879	- 33	3.91	- 0.13
1984	10.0	0.0	899	- 13	4.29	+0.25
1985	9.2	-0.6	885	- 27	3.95	- 0.09
1986	9.1	-0.7	992	+ 80	4.14	+0.09
1987	9.5	-0.3	919	+ 7	3.74	- 0.31
1988	10.2	+0.4	923	+ 9	4.05	0.00
1989	10.9	+1.1	814	- 98	4.80	+0.75
1990	11.1	+1.3	838	- 74	4.71	+0.66

* The average periods used are as follows:

Rainfall		Air temperature and daily sunshine	
Years	Average period	Years	Average period
1916-1976	1916-1950	1916-1962	1921-1950
1977 onwards	1941-1970	1963-1973	1931-1960
		1974-1984	1941-1970
		1985 onwards	1951-1980

Appendix A

Instructions for Completion of Notification of Infectious Disease Log Sheet (Form WL)

1.   **WEEK NUMBER -**   Should correspond with the week number given to the OPCS Weekly Return Monitor Series. Weeks end on Friday. Please see list of week numbers on the inside cover of this pad, which complies with the International Standard for week numbering.

2.   **PAGE NUMBER -**   This is a key to identifying the notification. Start a new series of page numbers each week.

3.   **WEEKLY MEASLES , MUMPS AND RUBELLA SUMMARIES -**   These should be completed at the end of the week. If no measles, mumps or rubella notifications, enter '0' in Total boxes and leave remaining boxes blank.

4.   **DISEASE NOTIFICATION LOG:**
     (a) Case No. -
        (Cols 1 - 2)

Preprinted - in conjunction with the Week and Page number identifies the notification for possible late correction or further enquiries.

     (b) Disease code -
        (Cols 3 - 4)

Code	Disease	
03	Whooping cough	
04	Scarlet fever	
06	Malaria	These diseases require
07	Ophthalmia neonatorum	no entry in columns 10 - 11
08	Tetanus	
09	Leptospirosis	
12	Meningococcal septicaemia (without meningitis)	

Code	Disease	
02	Dysentery	
05	Viral hepatitis	
20	Typhoid fever	
21	Paratyphoid fever	These diseases require
22	Food poisoning	an entry in columns 10 - 11
23	Tuberculosis	
24	Meningitis	
25	Acute poliomyelitis	
26	Acute encephalitis	

Code	Disease	
50	Cholera	
51	Plague	These diseases require
52	Anthrax	no entry in columns 10-11.
53	Diphtheria	Entries should be entered
54	Smallpox	in RED to indicate rare disease
55	Yellow fever	
56	Typhus	When recording typhus
57	Relapsing fever	please state the type on
58	Rabies	reverse of form WL
59	Viral haemorrhagic fever	

     (c) Sex -
        (Col 5)

1   Males
2   Females

     (d) Age in years -
        (Cols 6 - 7)

00   age under 1 year
01-98   age 01 to 98 (use 98 for age 98 and over)
99   age unknown

Appendix A - *continued*

(e) Age in months if
  age under one year
  (Cols 8 - 9)

Should be used only when age is under I year
(Please enter 00 in columns 6 and 7)

00	age under 1 month
01	1 month and under 2 months
02	2 months and under 3 months
03	3 months and under 4 months
04	4 months and under 5 months
05	5 months and under 6 months
06	6 months and under 7 months
07	7 months and under 8 months
08	8 months and under 9 months
09	9 months and under 10 months
10	10 months and under 11 months
11	11 months and under 1 year

(f) Specificity code - Use with disease codes 02, 05 and 20-26 as follows:-

(Cols 10 - 11) **Disease**   **Specificity code**

02 Dysentery

01 Presumed contracted abroad

02 Presumed contracted in GB

03 Not known where contracted

05 Viral hepatitis

01 Thought or known to be due to hepatitis A, presumed contracted abroad

02 Thought or known to be due to hepatitis A, presumed contracted in GB

03 Thought or known to be due to hepatitis A, not known where contracted

04 Thought or known to be due to hepatitis B, presumed contracted abroad

05 Thought or known to be due to hepatitis B, presumed contracted in GB

06 Thought or known to be due to hepatitis B, not known where contracted

07 Known to be hepatitis A negative and hepatitis B negative and no other cause known ('non A - non B'), presumed contracted abroad

08 Known to be hepatitis A negative and hepatitis B negative and no other cause known ('non A - non B'), presumed contracted in GB

65

Appendix A - *continued*

(f) **Specificity code** - Use with disease codes 02, 05 and 20-26 as follows:-

(Cols 10 - 11)	Disease		Specificity code

05 Viral hepatitis (cont'd)

- 09 Known to be hepatitis A negative and hepatitis B negative and no other cause known ('non A - non B'), not known where contracted
- 10 Other cause / cause not known, presumed contracted abroad
- 11 Other cause / cause not known, presumed contracted in GB
- 12 Other cause / cause not known, not known where contracted

20 Typhoid fever

- 01 Presumed contracted abroad
- 02 Presumed contracted in GB
- 03 Not known where contracted

21 Paratyphoid fever

- 01 Presumed contracted abroad
- 02 Presumed contracted in GB
- 03 Not known where contracted

22 Food poisoning

- 01 Formally notified, presumed contracted abroad
- 02 Formally notified, presumed contracted in GB
- 03 Formally notified, not known where contracted
- 04 Ascertained by other means, presumed contracted abroad
- 05 Ascertained by other means, presumed contracted in GB
- 06 Ascertained by other means, not known where contracted

23 Tuberculosis

- 01 Pulmonary lesion (with or without mediastinal nodes and / or pleural effusion)
- 02 Mediastinal nodes and / or a pleural effusion without a pulmonary lesion
- 03 Meningitis with or without "other forms" (except items in 1 and 2)
- 04 "Other forms" only (except meningitis and items in 1 and 2)

Appendix A - *continued*

(f) **Specificity code -** Use with disease codes 02, 05 and 20-26 as follows:-

(Cols 10 - 11)	<u>Disease</u>	<u>Specificity code</u>
	23 Tuberculosis (cont'd)	05 Items in both 1 and 3
		06 Items in both 1 and 4
		07 Items in both 2 and 3
		08 Items in both 2 and 4
		09 Chemoprophylaxis
	24 Meningitis	01 Meningococcal
		02 Pneumococcal
		03 Influenzal (Haemophilus influenzae)
		04 Viral
		05 Other specified
		06 Unspecified
	25 Acute poliomyelitis	01 Paralytic
		02 Non-paralytic
	26 Acute encephalitis	01 Infective
		02 Post-infectious

(g) **Correction -**
(Col 12)

The log should contain all original notifications. If the notification is corrected within the week, ie withdrawn, enter code X in this column. This procedure should not be used for correcting clerical errors. If these occur a line should be drawn through the incorrect entry and a new entry completed.

(h) **Supplementary information -**
(Col 13)

Not to be used at present.

(i) **For local use -**
(Cols 14 - 15)

These columns may be used for any purpose but the information will not be abstracted centrally by OPCS.

Weekly log sheet

LONDON BOROUGH / COUNTY DISTRICT ....

YEAR / WEEK ENDED ....

Week Number
Page Number

For OPCS use only

Measles	Case Number	Disease Code	Sex	Total	Under 1 mth	1 mnth	2 mnths	3 mnths	4 mnths	5 mnths	6 mnths	7 mnths	8 mnths	9 mnths	10 mnths	11 mnths	
	00	**01**	1(M)														↓
			2(F)														

	1 year	2 years	3 years	4 years	5 years	6 years	7 years	8 years	9 years	10-14 years	15-24 years	25 & over	Unknown
→													

Mumps	Case Number	Disease Code	Sex	Total	Under 1 year	1 year	2 years	3 years	4 years	5 years	6 years	7 years	8 years	9 years	10-14 years	15-24 years	25 & over	Unknown
	88	**10**	1(M)															
			2(F)															

Rubella	Case Number	Disease Code	Sex	Total	Under 1 year	1 year	2 years	3 years	4 years	5 years	6 years	7 years	8 years	9 years	10-14 years	15-24 years	25 & over	Unknown
	99	**11**	1(M)															
			2(F)															

Case Number		Disease Code		Sex	Age in Years		Age in Months *(If under 1 Year)*		Specificity Code		Correction	Supplementary Information	For Local Use		Case Number		Disease Code		Sex	Age in Years		Age in Months *(If under 1 Year)*		Specificity Code		Correction	Supplementary Information	For Local Use	
1	2	3	4	5	6	7	8	9	10	11	12	13	14	15	1	2	3	4	5	6	7	8	9	10	11	12	13	14	15
0	1														1	9													
0	2														2	0													
0	3														2	1													
0	4														2	2													
0	5														2	3													
0	6														2	4													
0	7														2	5													
0	8														2	6													
0	9														2	7													
1	0														2	8													
1	1														2	9													
1	2														3	0													
1	3														3	1													
1	4														3	2													
1	5														3	3													
1	6														3	4													
1	7														3	5													
1	8														3	6													

FORM WL   PLEASE POST THIS FORM IN THE ENVELOPE PROVIDED BY FRIDAY EVENING

YA19/4 9/91

68
Printed in the United Kingdom for HMSO
C7 9/92